CAMBRIDGE LIBRARY COLLECTION

Books of enduring scholarly value

History of Medicine

It is sobering to realise that as recently as the year in which On the Origin of Species was published, learned opinion was that diseases such as typhus and cholera were spread by a 'miasma', and suggestions that doctors should wash their hands before examining patients were greeted with mockery by the profession. The Cambridge Library Collection reissues milestone publications in the history of Western medicine as well as studies of other medical traditions. Its coverage ranges from Galen on anatomical procedures to Florence Nightingale's common-sense advice to nurses, and includes early research into genetics and mental health, colonial reports on tropical diseases, documents on public health and military medicine, and publications on spa culture and medicinal plants.

Notes on Military Hygiene for Officers of the Line

For those engaged in military conflict at the end of the nineteenth century, infection and disease were still as formidable enemies as the guns of an opposing army. Yet advances in sanitary science and understanding continued to help officers keep their troops in optimal fighting condition. After serving as an assistant surgeon for the Union Army during the American Civil War, Alfred Alexander Woodhull (1837–1921) began to publish on the topics of hygiene and sanitation, and how they related to military effectiveness. Arguably his most important publication, the present work was based on lectures he delivered at the US Infantry and Cavalry School. It covers such varied topics as the selection of men, uniform design, and the management of waste. First published in 1890, it was recommended as a textbook by the surgeon general of the time. Reissued here is the revised third edition, which appeared in 1904.

Notes on Military Hygiene for Officers of the Line

*A Syllabus of Lectures Formerly Delivered
at the U.S. Infantry and Cavalry School*

ALFRED A. WOODHULL

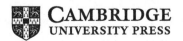

CAMBRIDGE
UNIVERSITY PRESS

CAMBRIDGE
UNIVERSITY PRESS

University Printing House, Cambridge, CB2 8BS, United Kingdom

Published in the United States of America by Cambridge University Press, New York

Cambridge University Press is part of the University of Cambridge.
It furthers the University's mission by disseminating knowledge in the pursuit of
education, learning and research at the highest international levels of excellence.

www.cambridge.org
Information on this title: www.cambridge.org/9781108069823

© in this compilation Cambridge University Press 2014

This edition first published 1904
This digitally printed version 2014

ISBN 978-1-108-06982-3 Paperback

NOTES

ON

MILITARY HYGIENE

FOR OFFICERS OF THE LINE.

A Syllabus of Lectures

FORMERLY DELIVERED AT

THE U. S. INFANTRY AND CAVALRY SCHOOL.

BY

ALFRED A. WOODHULL, A.M., M.D., LL.D. (*Princ.*)

*Colonel U. S. Army, Retired; Lately Colonel, Med. Dept. U. S. A.;
Lecturer on Personal Hygiene and on General
Sanitation, Princeton University.*

THIRD EDITION, REWRITTEN.

FIRST THOUSAND.

NEW YORK:

JOHN WILEY & SONS.

LONDON: CHAPMAN & HALL, LIMITED.

1904.

ROBERT DRUMMOND, PRINTER, NEW YORK.

PREFATORY NOTE.

THESE notes represent the essence of the lectures on Military Hygiene delivered to the class of 1889 at the Infantry and Cavalry School. The lectures were expansions of this syllabus, and were chiefly compilations with additions, comments, and illustrations from personal experience. Parkes's great work is the chief but not the only source whence the principles were drawn.

Originally prepared for the convenience of student officers, it has been thought that this abstract might be acceptable to officers of the line generally.

FORT LEAVENWORTH, May, 1890.

NOTE TO THE THIRD EDITION.

THE text has been changed when necessary to correspond with the present regulations for the army, and with the state of sanitary science.

The essay upon the care of troops in the field, especially in warm climates, was prepared for the second edition at the outbreak of the Spanish war. It is an expansion of parts of the body of the work, and to that extent duplicates what has been said in a fragmentary way. It is retained, revised and somewhat enlarged, under the belief that the subject merits this more connected discussion notwithstanding the required duplication. The aim throughout has been to stand in the place of a line officer anxious to take care of his command, and to find answers for his natural questions. As far as possible matters that belong exclusively to the medical staff have been omitted

PRINCETON, December, 1903.

CONTENTS.

NOTES ON MILITARY HYGIENE.

I.

THE SELECTION OF SOLDIERS.

Nature of Military Hygiene.

1. In general terms military hygiene means the care of troops. This duty is ever present, and it concerns line officers as they control the daily lives of men, and staff officers as they supply their food, their clothing, and their habitations.

2. It is of importance to soldiers because, removed from much independent action in relation to their own sanitary care, honesty requires they shall not be injured by the system imposed on them, and to the State because nothing is so costly as disease and nothing so remunerative as the outlay that augments health and thus increases the amount and value of the work done. (Parkes.)

General Physique.

3. The whole military fabric rests upon the physical character of the individuals composing it. The recruits must be trustworthy in physique before the military character can be developed, and extreme

care is necessary to avoid accepting blemished men who will break down under strain. Recruiting is, therefore, a serious duty, to be both conscientiously and intelligently performed.

4. It is not true, as sometimes assumed, that every full-grown man who supports himself by hard manual labor will make an efficient soldier; because all his senses may not be keen nor all his joints flexible, and although accustomed to vigorous work he may not be sound. Unsound men, enlisted on account of special skill as craftsmen, can never be depended on for the field and will certainly be absent in battle. When in doubt as to a recruit, reject.

5. Some allowance may be made for blemishes not affecting organic soundness that have originated in the service, in men who technically re-enlist, because their education in military matters and their habits of discipline compensate for some minor weaknesses. But all variations from the standard must be carefully noted on the enlistment papers. Blemished men who failed to re-enlist but seek to engage later are rarely acceptable. It usually means that they cannot succeed in civil life.

6. "An army raised without due regard to the choice of recruits was never yet made a good army by any length of service." (Vegetius, A.D. 300.)

Age of Recruits.

7. In peace, maximum for cavalry, 30 years; for all other arms, 35 years; minimum for musicians, 16 years; for all others, 18 years. No limit for subsequent enlistment.

8. Volunteers are accepted between 18 and 45,

but men were drafted in the Civil War only between
20 and 45. The unorganized militia are between 18
and 45, but no men of less than 20, and by preference
22, should ever be sent into the field.

Height and Weight.

9. Standards of height and weight are fixed by
regulation. Present minimum height, 5 ft. 4 in.
Maximum height for cavalry, 5 ft. 10 in.; for
all others as determined by relation to maximum
weight.

Cavalry, no minimum weight; cavalry and light
artillery, maximum, 165 pounds. For all others,
minimum weight, 128 pounds; maximum, 190
pounds. An exceptionally good recruit may be
accepted at 120 pounds, if completely filling all
other conditions.

10. Physiological relation between height and
weight, used as the standard for recruits, is: To include 5 ft. 7 in., 2 pounds to the inch and add 7
pounds for every inch above 5 ft. 7 in.

11. Application of rule for weight: Multiply the
whole height in inches by 2; multiply the difference
between 5 ft. 7 in. and a greater height by 5; add
the products.

Example: To find the normal weight of a man 5
ft. 10 in. 5 ft. 10 in. = 70 in.; $70 \times 2 = 140$; 5 ft.
7 in. = 67 in.; $70 - 67 = 3$; $3 \times 5 = 15$; $140 + 15 = 155$
= weight.

12. The maximum height for cavalry is fixed, and
it depends upon the maximum weight of 165 pounds
for light artillery and 190 pounds for all other
troops.

Example: 5 ft. 7 in. = 67 in.; 67×2 = 134; 190 − 134
= 56; 56 ÷ 7 = 8; 67 + 8 = 75 = 6 ft. 3 in. for foot
troops.

13. Present regulations permit the acceptance of
recruits a few pounds over or ten pounds below the
standard when active, vigorous, and healthy, with
firm muscles. But recruits under weight are to be
regarded with disfavor unless reduced by some manifestly temporary condition, and ten pounds less than
the standard for men under 5 ft. 7 in. involves
physiological risk. It is better that men, if muscular, should be over than under weight, but obese
men should be rejected whether short or tall.

14. The present minimum height, 5 ft. 4 in., is
merely a regulation that may be changed at any
time; but experience has shown that 5 ft. 2 in.
is practically the lowest limit for efficiency, and
when men less than 5 ft. have been accepted they
have been found to speedily break down as a class
from want of physical strength.

15. Tailors, bandsmen, school-teachers, and similar skilled men may be accepted if not more than
one-fourth inch below the minimum. Exceptions
as to over-height may be authorized at the War
Department; but exceedingly tall men serve only
an ornamental purpose, such as drum-majors.
They are seldom very serviceable in the ranks.
The best all-around soldiers are between 5 ft. 6
in. and 5 ft. 10 in.

Chest Capacity.

16. Chest capacity is determined by the factors of
chest measurement and chest mobility, and is an

important element in estimating vigor. The circumference of the chest should be measured at forced expiration and forced inspiration. The size at expiration is the more important, and it is that to which the designation of chest measurement is technically applied.

17. The official direction is to apply "a tape at the point of the shoulder-blade, when it will generally fall below the nipple." In actual practice the tape is generally applied in front just below the nipple, which brings it rather above the point of the shoulder-blade. Otherwise an oblique rather than a horizontal plane is described.

18. Chest mobility is the difference between the extremes of expiration and inspiration. The circumference at the nipple should be about one-half the height of the man, and, speaking generally, the more nearly the chest approaches a barrel in shape the better.

19. The capacity of the lungs increases with age to a certain period and with height and growth, so that men from 5 to 6 ft. high inspire from 174 to 262 in.

20. The physiological rule to determine the relation of chest capacity to height in recruits is: Between 5 ft. 4 in. and 5 ft. 7 in. the mean of the chest circumference ought to be 34 in., and there must be a chest mobility of 2 in., with *a minimum at expiration of* 32 *in.* Above 5 ft. 7 in. the mobility should be 2½ in., and for every inch of stature add one-half inch to chest measurement. For 6 ft. and more the mobility should be 3 in.

21. The physiological rule and the official rule formerly agreed substantially, but for a few years

past the regulation has established a lower standard and, further, has authorized the chest measurement—the circumference at forced expiration—to be 2 in. still less when the recruit is active, vigorous, and healthy. No recruit should be accepted who is not active, vigorous, and healthy, and officers are particularly warned against taking advantage of this further reduction.

22. Table showing the relation between height, weight, and chest capacity under the old and the existing standards.

(*Greenleaf, modified.*)

Height. Inches.	Weight. Pounds.	Chest measurement (at expiration). Old. Inches.	New. Inches.	Chest mobility. Inches.
64	128	32½	32	2
65	130	33	32	2
66	132	33½	32½	2
67	134	34	33	2
68	141	34	33¼	2½
69	148	34½	33½	2½
70	155	35	34	2½
71	162	35¼	34¼	2½
72	169	35¾	34¾	3
73	176	36¼	35¼	3

Minors.

23. All military experience is opposed to the enlistment of minors for active service, and, notwithstanding it is legal to enlist a minor above the age of 18 with his parents' consent, provided he is in all respects the equal of a man of 21, it rarely happens that such a lad responds to the tests of the field. This proviso is extremely important, and officers not insisting on this standard or not recognizing the physical deficiencies of a bright lad of 19 are liable to weaken the service by such enlistments.

24. Napoleon after Leipsic said: "I must have grown men; boys serve only to fill the hospitals and encumber the roadside."

25. In Egypt, in 1798, the 68th from Bombay was composed chiefly of boys. Fever broke out on their passage, they lost nearly half their number, and continued so sickly that they were re-embarked and sent back. But the 61st, over 900 strong, nearly all old soldiers, were sixteen weeks on board ship and landed with only one man sick. (It is probable, however, that the condition of the transports and the care exercised over the men had much to do with their health in both of these cases.)

26. In the Peninsular War, 1805–14, 300 men who had served five years were regarded more effective than a newly arrived regiment of 1000 recruits who were lads.

27. In the Mexican War, 1847, our medical officers constantly reported that the inferior physique, and especially the youth of the recruits, materially increased the sick and mortality lists.

28. In the Crimea, 1854–55, when notified that 2000 recruits were ready, Lord Raglan replied that "those last sent were so young and unformed that they fell victims to disease and were swept away like flies, so that he preferred to wait," rather than to have young lads sent out as soldiers.

29. Lord Hardinge says that "although no men were sent [to the Crimea] under 19 years of age, yet when sent out it was found that instead of being composed of bone and muscle they were almost gristle."

30. In General Roberts's march from Cabul to

Candahar in 1880 "it was the young soldiers who succumbed to its fatigues, while the old soldiers became hardier and stronger every day." The Franco-German experience coincides with all this.

31. The influence of age upon disability in the field during the Civil War has not been shown by authentic statistics, but the experience of all officers serving with troops then will confirm the general statement that very young men generally broke down first under exposure and hardship.

32. In peace, as well, the official reports show that below the age of 25 the rate of sickness very much exceeds the mean for the whole army.

33. Discussing the defectives in the Philippines, during and after the insurrection of 1899–1900, Birmingham ranks first "the immature youth. The number of undeveloped boys, ranging in age from 17 to 21, met with in the hospitals, whose only chance for life lay in building up their strength sufficiently to admit of their being put on the first transport sailing for home, was simply deplorable." Personal observation entirely agrees with this.

34. "A large majority of the men (or boys) invalided home from the Philippines were in their first or second year of service, and a great many were taken off transports, put in hospitals, and shipped home without doing a day's duty." (*Private letter.*)

35. "This general assent shows how wrong it is to expect any great and long-continued exercise of force from lads as young as 18 or 20, and the inevitable consequences of taxing them beyond their strength." (Marshall.)

36. *Per contra:* Young men are more easily trained and moulded than older men, especially for the cavalry, and when well led fight as well, as far as mere physical courage goes.

37. But as we cannot keep young soldiers several years in training, and as large bodies of troops will only be raised for sudden war, men not absolutely mature must be rejected, for the most effective armies have always been those where the youngest men were 22.

38. If battalions of military apprentices should be authorized, as once proposed, to be trained and kept occupied in practical military work at home, they should completely replace the minors now unwisely enlisted in the line and develop into excellent soldiers.

Growth and Development.

39. Growth "is the gradual increase to full size by the addition of matter," and development "is the advancement of an organized being from one stage to another toward a more complete state." Because a man has acquired his growth, it by no means follows that he is fully developed. Physical maturity does not occur until nearly the twenty-fifth year, and a man less than 22, and especially one not yet 20, is very liable to break down under the conditions of military life.

40. The skeleton is designed to enclose, support, and defend the important organs of life, and for locomotion. The bones which make it up arise from separate centres and coalesce so slowly that some of them are not consolidated until the twenty-fifth year.

41. The weakest part of the spine is that of its greatest curve, at the "hollow of the back," and here the circle of the body, the waist, is least. Here the jar of a false step, the fatigue of drills and marches, and the early aching in fevers are most severely felt.

42. The sacrum and hip-bones together form a buttress and arches adapted to support weights, and upon them men can best sustain burdens, whether in military or civil life. These are consolidated at the 25th year.

43. Other physiological considerations in connection with the young soldier are the growth of the bones and muscles in relation to each other; for the muscles, or flesh, by whose contractions physical movements are made, are attached by their extremities, and sometimes along part of their length to the bones. Large and powerful muscles require proportionately large and powerful bones, and well-developed points, ridges, and prominences upon these for their attachment.

44. The bones become thicker, the joints stronger, and the shoulders broader from the 20th to 25th year, the maximum height is barely attained at 25, and the muscles gradually develop in size and strength up to 30th year.

Effect of Pressure upon Contents of Chest.

45. One important function of the skeleton is to enclose and protect the heart and lungs in the cavity of the chest; notwithstanding which these organs suffer more in the recruit whatever his age, but

especially in the young, than in the seasoned soldier.

46. "Next to the inspiration of bad air, the imperfect or continuously obstructed expansion of the chest tends more than any cause we know of to bring about diseases of the heart and lungs." (Aitken.)

47. Pressure before or behind tends to "set" growing bones in an unnatural direction, or to cripple the lungs by confining the chest-walls, and even canteen and haversack straps may press upon the immature recruit to his harm.

48. Nevertheless, in the field the soldier must carry packs of some sort, which, especially when ill adjusted, tend materially to derange the contained chest organs.

Growth and Development of Lungs and Heart.

49. It is indispensable that these organs shall be sound and well developed. Both of them increase in size and weight, especially between the 14th and 25th years, unless crippled by an insufficient bony case, as sometimes occurs to the lungs.

50. The greatest proportionate growth of the heart is during the change known as the accession of puberty, when it nearly doubles its size. If that occupies five years the heart-increase each year is one-fifth; but if it occurs in one year, the growth is so much more rapid that the heart may become weak out of all proportion to its size. A heart that grows in one year three times as much as in the preceding year is almost necessarily weak. Hence a recruit with a so rapidly developed heart is not acceptable for continuous labor. The heart

continues to increase in size after puberty, and its greatest amount of growth is from the 18th to 25th year.

51. "The greatest strain is thrown on the heart throughout adolescence to adult age, and a very constant group of symptoms indicates the cardiac failure that must be looked for in overworked recruits." (Aitken.)

52. This heart-strain from excessive fatigue in those who have grown rapidly and who have deficient reserve energy is apt to lead to heart-failure under unwonted exertion and in emergencies. It is this liability in the young soldier, whether he has grown rapidly or not, that is one of the most serious objections to immature levies.

Effect of Injudicious Drill upon Recruits.

53. Military drill is intended (1) to instruct the man in certain movements for his greater efficiency as a soldier acting with others, and (2) to develop a power of physical endurance. A young recruit cannot keep pace with a full-grown and completely trained man in the ranks, mainly because his heart and blood-vessels are not fully developed nor specially accustomed to the work. Failure usually arises from attempting too much at the outset; and with excessive work at the begininng, or with a sudden increase, as in forced marches, these youths rapidly break down.

54. Drill must begin within the powers of endurance of the recruit, and the young soldier, usually keeping up too long from pride, should be encouraged to fall out of ranks when distressed. "The

throb of the heart and the swell of the arteries and veins must be allowed to subside and settle down completely, so that the lungs may resume their peaceful action of easy breathing, before any further drill exertion is attempted." (Aitken.) If his breathing does not gradually improve, or if the man's weight continues to decline, he should without further delay be referred to the medical officer for examination.

55. Treatment in such cases cannot be hurried. To take a young soldier into hospital for a week or two only gives temporary ease. No medicine is a substitute for strength, and it may require six months for the heart to recover from one strain. The same symptoms will recur again and again under similar circumstances, until the condition is outgrown by development maturing, or the heart is permanently damaged.

Influence of Age and Height.

56. But while immature men should not be accepted, neither are too old men good recruits. The regulation limit in peace of 35 (30 for cavalry) is the extreme under ordinary conditions. As long as they are physically sound, recruits are legally acceptable in war under 45, but as they approach 30 common laborers are liable to become stiffened in body and mentally dulled, and few men of middle age enlisting for the first time are able to endure the strain of the field. In the Spanish war men from the coal-mines of Pennsylvania, although used to hard labor, proved as a class physically most unacceptable recruits.

57. Under existing orders very tall men are practically excluded. Were there no regulation, tall *young* men would be objectionable because their height is often gained at the expense of bulk or of the vigor of heart and lungs. A soldier is a machine of two parts; legs and arms offensive, chest and abdomen vital. Within the latter is generated the power that makes the former available.

58. An ill-proportioned tall man is undesirable. If analysis of such an applicant shows that he is tall by virtue of his legs and neck alone, remember that he will become tired sooner, partly because his muscles are relatively smaller and the levers they operate (the bones) are longer than those of shorter men, and partly because probably less vital force is generated in the less capacious chest and abdomen.

59. That the strongest army is the best army is a saying as old as the Romans, and properly interpreted it is true. Other things being equal, those with the most endurance are the best soldiers. Certainly the troops that march best are the most efficient, and are those on whom generals must depend. The marching qualities of Ord's infantry made Appomattox possible.

Examination of Recruits.

60. It is a recruiting officer's duty to select critically and accept only those who will probably become strong and active soldiers. The test of mere numbers is a very poor one to determine the efficiency of a recruiting officer, for they are true maxims "that an army consists of the bayonets in the field, not the names on the muster-roll," "nothing is so

expensive as an unhealthy military force" (Farr), and "it is of much more importance that a soldier should be strong than that he should be tall." (Vegetius.)

61. The recruiting regulations carefully followed are a safe and explicit guide. But there is a constant tendency to disregard their minutiæ, under the feeling that, apart from obscure diseases, any officer accustomed to soldiers can recognize a good recruit at sight. Therefore, disregarding morbid conditions only discoverable by a physician, special attention is invited to the following points.

62. The physiological requirements of height, weight, and chest capacity should be carefully observed, because they are based upon natural laws that cannot be disregarded with impunity.

63. No precise standard of intelligence can be formulated, but care must be taken to exclude men not capable of appreciating the improved weapons and the more responsible duties of the modern soldier. "The development of the head and the symmetry of its proportion should be as carefully insisted upon as with other organs and regions." (Crawford.) Examine the head with the fingers carefully, and for any depression not certainly natural, for any serious scar, or for any sensitive spot, reject. Such men invariably break down under exposure to heat or to great fatigue.

64. All lank, slight, puny men with contracted figure—men technically termed as of "poor physique"—should be set aside, for there is no class that furnishes so large a proportion to the hospital and the guard-house as this. "Another class hav-

ing neither apparent disease nor well-characterized
physical or moral defect is equally objectionable;
there is a 'something' about them [which may well
be termed want of aptitude] which satisfies an ex-
pert that they will make either indifferent or bad
soldiers." (Greenleaf.) In all cases of doubt, reject. It is sheer waste for the government to take
care of incompetents. The army is neither a reform-
atory nor an almshouse.

65. The utmost care should be had to exclude men
likely to be intemperate, for the intolerable nuisance that drunkards are within the service warrants
the risk of occasionally rejecting a sober man rather
than to accept those who constantly make trouble
in peace and who cannot be depended on in war.

66. When a recruiting officer has merely an un-
trained civil physician, one not practically familiar
with military·life, to assist him, he must depend in
great measure upon his own observation and judgment. Many a first-class life-insurance risk would
be utterly worthless as a soldier.

67. A summary of the general qualifications is:
"A tolerably just proportion between the different
parts of the trunk and members, a well-shaped
head, thick hair, a countenance expressive of health,
with a lively eye, skin not too white, lips red, teeth
white and in good condition, voice strong, skin firm,
chest well-formed, belly lank, organs of generation
well developed, limbs muscular, feet arched and of
moderate length, hands large."

68. Sound opposing teeth to chew well the difficult food of the field are necessary. At the least
there must be two good grinders opposite each

other on each side. Unmasticated food leads to intestinal disease, and carious teeth, especially in early life, mark a feeble constitution easily undermined.

69. Should the pulse at either wrist drop a beat at intervals, either before or after exercise, reject.

70. Vision of each eye as tried by test-cards must be acute. Each eye in turn should be covered by card-board, not by the hand.

71. Hearing of each ear must easily distinguish ordinary conversation at fifty feet. Unilateral deafness is only distinguishable by carefully closing each ear in succession by pressure, and is disqualifying.

72. While all joints must be mobile, special pains should be paid to the right thumb and forefinger, so important in handling arms. The thumb, acting in opposition to the rest of the hand, is the characteristic distinction between man and the quadrumana. It affords the grasp which makes weaving, building fires, and the use of weapons possible. (Whitehead.) Strength and mobility in the thumb are indispensable.

73. The testicles must be handled, and if either is sensitive or both have dwindled, reject.

74. For visible veins of the ankle, behind the knee, or on the thigh, reject when they are really large and multiple. A few inconspicuous veins do not disqualify spare men.

75. Determine the soundness of the lower limbs by vigorous exercise. Observe keenly that each limb does its full share of work. Count silently the number of hops with each leg in passing twice over a given distance; should they differ, there is weakness or stiffness.

76. Flatfootedness, a peculiar dread of many recruiting officers, and thus leading to the occasional
rejection of fair men, is rarely seen among the whites
of this country. In the disqualifying flat foot the
inner ankle is very prominent and lower than usual;
there is a hollow of greater or less extent below the
outer ankle; the foot is not well arched, and is
broader at the ankle than near the toes; the inner
side is flat and occasionally convex, and when placed
on the ground the finger cannot be introduced
beneath the sole; the weight of the body rests on
the inner side of the sole, and the ordinary motions
of the ankle are impaired.

77. For bunions, large or recently inflamed, reject.
A tightly fitting shoe will at once disqualify with them.
Corns on the sole are mischievous, and when under
the base of the great toe condemn. Numerous corns
may cripple the foot for prolonged walking.

78. Fœtid perspiration of the feet is intolerable
in a squad-room. A recruit so afflicted should not
be accepted and if inadvertently enlisted should be
discharged. That is a disease, and is distinct from
want of cleanliness.

79. A toe, usually the second, sometimes is stiffened at right angles so that the nail touches the
ground. Reject, because sand will work under the
nail and cause inflammation. This is known as
"hammer-toe," or "walking on the nail." Occasionally one toe, permanently displaced by a tight
shoe in youth, will overlap another. That is disqualifying, notwithstanding the man may not limp
when examined.

80. Unsightly markings are disqualifying, because they lead to rude and vexatious jests.

81. The preceding points are those most apt to be overlooked by inexperienced officers, and stress is laid upon their importance in securing sound men.

82. Vaccination as a practical immunity against smallpox should be carefully but not too frequently practised. Thorough vaccination in infancy repeated at the age of 14–16 will generally protect, but every recruit should be presented for examination as soon as he reaches a proper station.

General Considerations.

83. In war, especially under a general enrolment, men with minor physical blemishes may properly be accepted provided their general health is sound, but every variation from the standard in peace or war should be carefully noted on the descriptive lists.

84. In raising new troops when it is possible to select, for sharp and immediate active service take town-bred men. If a year or two can be had in which to train them, take country-bred men.

85. Open-air military life is physical promotion to city men accustomed to irregular hours, unwholesome meals, and poorly ventilated rooms. They are the survivors from the contagious diseases, which nearly all of them have had, and their minds are much more active for the reception of new ideas of drill and discipline, although not always particularly docile. They must be more carefully scrutinized for the physical stains of vice.

86. To young men from the country the irregular

and sometimes scanty meals, broken rest, necessity for prompt and exact action, and above all the certainty of acquiring such diseases as measles, whooping-cough, and mumps, which town boys always have in childhood, are very exhausting. After a year's training country recruits are more valuable, generally showing more endurance when seasoned.

87. But never be satisfied with minors, and always give preference to men of mature physique. In a volunteer regiment that preserved excellent health under particularly unfavorable conditions in one of the large camps of 1898, the men were well beyond minority and were thoroughly matured. They had been carefully selected by one of their officers who had been an intelligent sergeant in the army, and they displayed remarkable resistance to very pernicious surroundings.

88. After muster-in all volunteers should be detained for a short time in a special camp, to weed out the inadvertently-accepted imperfect men. As the effectiveness of any command depends on vigor rather than numbers, all frail men should then be discharged and the civil origin of their pre-existing disabilities be clearly noted on their papers. Even at that date it is much better to discharge than to retain doubtful men.

89. Even with seasoned troops special examination should also exclude the temporarily weak from any serious march or expedition, due allowance being made for malingering. A column intended for vigorous service should be free from men who would limit its action. Such temporary exempts may always be usefully employed at the base.

90. Measles is a particularly serious camp disease, always to be anticipated in newly raised commands, especially ravaging those from the rural districts. In the Civil War there were 67,700 cases with 4200 deaths among white troops and 8555 cases with 933 deaths among colored troops in the Union Army. (See par. 788.)

91. Typhoid fever (which see later) is always to be found among large bodies of recruits, where it will spread unless competent medical advice as to its prevention is carefully followed. Enormous camps of new troops as sometimes organized are hurtful, because of their tendency to propagate disease.

92. It would be a mistake to accept militia commands as a whole, even for a limited time, without close individual scrutiny. Usually their physical requirements for membership are very light, and their acquaintance with drill does not compensate for a low average in years and physique.

93. The matter of recruiting is thus dwelt upon because it is the foundation upon which the whole military organization rests. It is impossible to have an efficient army without carefully selected men. And after enlistment an equal duty rests upon company officers to see that these men are not injured by their new surroundings.

Comparison between Sickness and Violence.

94. Very little sickness is spontaneous, and with an army of sound men there is no good reason why there should be much loss of duty from disease. When company officers study for themselves the problems of ventilation, of food, of the healthfulness

of camps, of water-supply, of the disposal of excreta, when they concern themselves with soldiers as physiological agents, the army will be prepared for the highest exhibition of sustained action.

95. As would be supposed, in peace, when casualties by violence are few, the disability by disease is out of all proportion to that by injury. But in war also deaths from sickness, quite independently of that sickness which is recovered from or which leads to discharge without immediate loss of life, outnumber many fold those from battle. Unlike in peace, very many of the disease-causes of war are unavoidable.

96. In the Mexican War, of the regular force 73 officers and 862 men, total 935, were killed or died of wounds, and 85 officers and 4629 men, total 4714, died of disease in the field, or rather less than 1 to 5.

Of the volunteers 1549 officers and men died by violence and 10,986 by disease, or a little less than 1 to 7.

97. During the Rebellion 99,183 white troops died from the casualties of battle and 171,806 from disease, or nearly 1 to 2; while for colored troops it was 3417 by violence and 29,963 by disease, or 1 to 8.7.

98. The Santiago campaign of 1898, successful in the direct collision, culminated in the virtual dissolution, from disease, of the invading corps as a further aggressive force. The Philippine insurrection of 1899 filled the hospitals with the seriously sick, while the casualties of action were moderate.

In the Philippines, in the eighteen months following July 1, 1898, 36 officers and 489 men, total 525, were killed in action or died of wounds, and 16 officers and 693 men, total 809, died of disease. This is as 1 to 1.7. These were exclusive of 587 discharged

for disability and 1901 transferred to the United
States incapacitated, both groups including all
causes. The non-fatal wounds were 1767. The
number constantly sick was enormously in excess of
those off duty from wounds. Harrington, including
the statistics of the entire force at all places for the
Cuban and the Philippine campaigns for the year
ending April 30, 1899, states that 968 men were
killed or died of wounds, injuries, or accidents (not
all, therefore, in battle) and 5438 died from disease,
or 1 to 5.6. In these figures "men" probably includes officers.

99. The German army in the war of 1870–71 is
the only one known to have kept its mortality from
disease below that from battle. This probably depended upon the shortness of the war, the rapid succession of battles, the trained troops, and presumably upon its exact discipline being exerted for the
care of the men as well as in other directions.

100. But the amount of disease, rather than the
number of deaths, is the measure of physical inca-
pacity for an army. It matters very little what the
particular cause of the unfitness may be at any one
time, as long as so many men are then unfit for duty.
The actual and the probable sick reports combined
restrain a command, by interfering with its mobility
and weakening its fighting power. By the probable
sick report is meant such a state of health or endurance that, while it allows a command to do a certain
form of duty, say in garrison, might not permit it to
keep the field or to undergo peculiar hardships.
The influence of line officers, and especially of commanding officers, is very potent here.

II.

MILITARY CLOTHING.

Its Object.

101. As the non-essentials of dress are usually both valueless and inconvenient in war, the clothing that the soldier is compelled to wear should be simple and suited to his arduous work.

102. The essential object of all clothing is the protection of the person from extremes of temperature by conserving bodily heat in cold weather and preventing suffering from either solar heat or that generated by exercise.

103. A secondary object of military clothing is to encourage proper professional pride in the soldier, to aid in determining his place in the army, and to render him inconspicuous to the enemy.

Distinctive Markings.

104. Each arm should be distinguished, as at present, by its appropriate dress, and in large commands the divisions may conveniently be identified by corps badges.

105. Corps badges are devices systematized and attached to the cap; *e.g.*, a Maltese cross, a trefoil, a diamond in cloth, as the device for the corps; then those of the first division would be red, of the second white, of the third blue on a white ground, the fourth

24

orange. These should be undiscernible to the foe, but serve both for identification and as a sign of comradeship within the army.

106. There is a constant temptation with new troops to wear some conspicuous mark of regimental significance, whose ultimate effect is to draw fire. This should never be permitted.

107. Regimental facings are sometimes pressed in the interest of regimental *esprit*. Good results would follow with good troops. But a minor obstacle is that of cost, and a serious one that of supply. In the Crimea the British suffered severely in attempting to keep up distinctive regimental clothing, and until it was abandoned the men were not sufficiently clad.

108. Our State troops will probably long maintain showy dress uniforms for purposes of display. But their fighting clothing, the undress, should be uniform with that of the United States for convenience of administration.

Color.

109. Color is a military and a physiological factor in clothing. Military garments should be neutral in tint. Gray and drab are the best colors, and next a light butternut dye.

110. The order in which colors draw fire is red, white, black or dark blue, light blue, butternut, dust-gray, and drab. Scarlet tells with great effect upon the wearer, and certain so-called zouave regiments certainly left some dead upon the field that would have been spared in a plainer dress. The old-fashioned white cross-belts have had many

victims. The same is true of the white shoulder-straps lately in use on khaki coats, which were conspicuous marks between which to aim.

111. Gray varies considerably in shade, so that at one end of the scale it differs but little from light blue. But in large masses, dust-gray (khaki) and drab are the most nearly invisible. This is particularly true in arid countries and among forests. The stain of ordinary soil is less marked upon it.

112. Therefore, for service, as exposed to long-range firearms, the least conspicuous the dress the better.

113. The color of full-dress uniform has no hygienic quality, except in tropical climates, where it should approach as nearly as possible to white.

114. Protection against the sun's rays depends entirely upon color, irrespective of texture. Color does not influence bodily heat, nor the external temperature except as directly derived from the sun. White absorbs the least heat, and is therefore the coolest; black the most, and is the warmest; and blue is next to black. A thin white cotton tissue worn over a dark cloth coat will reduce the temperature by 12.6° F. in very hot sun's rays.

115. The absorption of odor depends partly upon texture, in proportion to the hygroscopic power of the material, and partly upon color. Black absorbs odors the most, blue next, white least. Dark colors, therefore, should not be worn by those associated with the sick.

MATERIALS.

116. Clothing creates no heat. Depending upon color, not upon texture, it absorbs the direct solar rays. Further than that it is hot or cool just as it retains the heat of the body or allows it to escape.

Cotton and Linen.

117. Both cotton and linen conduct heat rapidly, and neither absorbs water well; so the perspiration passes directly through to the outer surface, where it evaporates.

118. The heat generated by bodily exercise is reduced by the evaporation of the sensible perspiration. When the exertion ceases the generation of heat is reduced, but the flow of perspiration persists for the time, so that, where its rapid evaporation continues, the consequent chilling of the body is liable to be followed by sickness.

119. As cotton and linen, even when dry, conduct heat away from the body rapidly, and as they speedily become drenched by perspiration, this rapid evaporation proceeds practically unchecked. They are therefore unsuited for ordinary military clothing, and are positively dangerous for men liable to violent exertion followed by sudden rest.

120. A special weave of linen is now on the market, for which it is claimed that so much air is entangled in an open mesh as to obviate some of these disadvantages.

121. Nevertheless, when the temperature of the air in the shade approaches for considerable periods the normal heat of the body (100° F.), the system

becomes enervated and the clothing should not add
to that embarrassment, as heavy wool, formerly
worn universally, would. Therefore a white duck
sack-coat and trousers may be worn at home in
summer, in extreme southern latitudes, when authorized by the department commander. This pre-
supposes wearing a light woollen undershirt also.

122. So in tropical climates cotton duck, white
in garrison and olive-drab in the field, guarded
by mixed woollen underwear, is appropriate. But
starched cotton and linen are nearly impermeable
to air and are very hot, until broken down by perspiration. Cotton is cheap and is very durable.

123. White cotton outer clothing is authorized on
sanitary grounds for Hospital Corps soldiers doing
ward duty at any station.

Wool.

124. Wool conducts heat badly and absorbs
water freely in two ways. The water permeates
and distends the fibres of the wool (hygroscopic
water) and lies between the fibres (water of inter-
position). In relation to cotton or linen, wool absorbs hygroscopically at least double in proportion
to its weight and quadruple in proportion to its
surface.

125. By absorbing the perspiration, wool counter-
acts the evaporation that persists after excessive
exercise. Dry woollen clothing condenses the vapor
from the surface of the body and gives out much
heat that had become latent when the water of the
body was vaporized (insensible perspiration).

126. While dry wool is of course better than wet

woollen clothing, it is rare that woollen clothes become saturated with bodily moisture; and even when they do, they may be partly dried by wringing, and thus become useful for further condensation and absorption.

127. Wool is not easily penetrated by cold winds, and its quality of non-conduction makes it useful in cold and oppressive in warm climaves.

128. The chief disadvantage of woollen clothing, where the climate is suitable, is the difficulty in washing it. Badly washed, it shrinks in the fibre, and the whole after a time becomes smaller, harder, and probably less absorbent. This is the bar to the issue of pure woollen underclothing for the field. The remedy is the admixture of about 30 per cent. of cotton, making the so-called merino.

129. To wash woollens they should be placed in hot soap-suds and moved about freely; they should then be plunged in cold water, and when the soap has disappeared should be hung up without wringing. Woollens should never be rubbed nor wrung. (Parkes.) Or put the woollens into water by themselves; do not rub soap on them, but have it abundant in the water; move them about freely for cleansing; rinse them well, without rubbing, in clean water of the same temperature; hang them to dry without rubbing or wringing, but be careful to stretch them a little while drying. The soap should be free from excess of alkali, which injures the wool by its action on the natural fat.

130. Whatever foundation there may be for the older opinion that an all-wool dress is a partial preventive against the malarial poison probably de-

pends on the equable temperature thus maintained, which adds to the resistance of the system, and to the mechanical guard that its greater bulk presents against the mosquito.

131. Tests for woollen cloth: When held against the light, it should show a uniform texture, free from holes; folded and suddenly stretched, it should give a clear ringing note; it should resist well when violently stretched; to the touch the texture must be smooth and soft; to the eye it should be close and free from straggly hair. The heavier it is to the size, the better.

132. Shoddy is old, used, and worked-over wool and cloth. It is often mixed with fresh wool, to the detriment of the latter, and is most easily detected by the tearing power. This adulteration prevails under the greed of war, and should be carefully inspected against.

133. Serge is a species of worsted that has the advantage of lightness combined with the good qualities of the lesser woollens. Closely woven cloth, whatever the material, takes up dust less readily and parts with it more easily than that of loose texture.

Other Materials.

134. Other materials used as auxiliary clothing are leather, canvas, india-rubber, and oiled cloth.

135. Leather when properly tanned is practically impervious to the wind and is very warm; but it is only fit for rainless climates, except as foot-gear.

136. Canvas sheds water and is an excellent non-conductor of heat, and lined with wool it is admirable against cold.

137. "Slickers," made by thoroughly washing canvas and soaking it with raw oil slowly dried in the sun, are admirable against rain, although not officially recognized.

138. India-rubber has a temporary but invaluable use against rain, but cannot be worn persistently on account of its retaining the bodily heat and the perspiration. It loses its elasticity in very cold climates and becomes too distensible in very warm ones. It ultimately rots by the absorption of oxygen. As a water-proof sheet to place on the ground it is of great value.

139. India-rubber may be replaced by the application to ordinary clothing of a water-proofing process devised by Captain Munson, Medical Department. Fabrics thus treated do not lose their shape; will shed water under heavy rain for several hours; their ventilation is unimpaired; and there is no sense of bearing about wet clothing. Animal materials respond to the process better than those that are vegetable, but the latter can be made to shed water. This quality is destroyed by boiling water or strongly alkaline soap, but it may be renewed by re-immersion in the water-proof bath.

Head Covering.

140. The ideal military hat should protect against heat, cold, rain, and the glare of the sun. It should be attractive on parade, convenient under arms, and useful in bivouac. Such has not yet been found in any service.

141. The newly adopted cap for garrison use is of cloth, three and a half inches deep, with an over-

hanging top. It should afford an air space above, but it gives no protection below the line of contact. Its color depends upon the duty. It would seem practicable to use separate covers with a common frame.

142. A service hat of drab felt with a moderately broad brim is now issued for drills, marches, and the field. It is tolerably high in the crown, and when this is drawn to a peak, which at present is forbidden, the air space is increased and rain-water is shed. It is substantially the equivalent of the older campaign hat, which, although not perfect, proved very acceptable in the field in all climates.

143. The white or drab cork helmet is a comfortable protection against the fierce sun, but it is unfit for cold seasons and is too inflexible for the field. Properly made, it is well ventilated.

144. An ordinary sportsman's hat, with specially high crown for the tropics, double peak, and folding flaps, as evolved by hunters, would fulfil the requirements of open-air life. Of neutral color it may be decorated if desired, but it should not be ornamented for the field. For hot weather it should be of light canvas, and for cold seasons be lined. This would be light in weight, not in the way of the man's weapons, it would be a shelter by day and a protection by night in the field, and it has stood the test of much rough usage with the reputation of comfort and durability.

145. In the tropics the nape of the neck must be guarded against the sun by a peak at the rear, the crown should always be high and well-ventilated, and a contained piece of wet muslin assists against

heat-stroke. A stiff hat in hot climates should be held away from the head by an inner band for ventilation.

Coats.

146. The closely fitting dress-coat, the most unhygienic and therefore unmilitary article of a soldier's dress, has been discontinued for some years for the Hospital Corps, and lately has been abandoned by the rest of the army. Nothing should ever lead to its revival. It compressed the chest and interfered with its expansion, and it restrained the soldier from the vigorous exertion to which his training is directed.

147. Dress-coats will doubtless be retained for the time by State troops purely for purposes of display and attraction, but inspecting officers should always condemn those that are tight and should discourage their being taken into the field. When mustered into the United States service, that part of the uniform should be rejected.

148. Tight collars, whether of coats or shirts, disturb the blood-supply of the head, affect vision, and may lead to serious consequences. The neck should be free from the least compression.

149. The dark-blue sack-coat, designated for purposes of ceremony, should always fit loosely. The inevitable tendency of the tailors will be to make it more and more snug, and company officers should guard against that on principle. It should never be taken to the tropics nor worn in the South at home.

150. The present service coat, of woollen or cotton, is wisely required to be five inches in excess of the

chest measurement. It contains two outside pockets above and two below the waist-line, and promises to be very serviceable. Except that there is no belt between the body and the skirt upon which the waist-belt of the accoutrements may fit accurately, this closely resembles in form, and substantially in principle, the plan of the hunting-shirt, the typical military dress, that has been advocated for years. It should always be loose enough for extra shirts to be worn.

151. The objection formerly made to a loosely fitting dress was to call it slouchy. That has no real force, for no man held in position by his clothes is either very vigorous or soldierly. Setting up, not tight clothing, makes the martial figure. All clothing should be neatly cut, but none should limit the freest muscular action.

Shirts.

152. A knit woollen undershirt, which sometimes is unbearable by delicate skins, and, formerly at least, was too short, is issued. The later issues are better. It should be one-third cotton for ordinary issue and in three grades of thickness. A soldier should be allowed to draw two sizes, to wear one over the other if necessary. In hot climates this should be two-thirds cotton.

153. An overshirt of flannel is now issued. This has a rolling collar and breast-pockets, is reasonably full, and may be worn without the coat on fatigue. It approaches the hunting-shirt and is comfortable and useful. It should be issued in three grades and

many sizes, with and without collars, for two or more to be worn together.

154. Animal heat is best conserved by several superimposed similar garments, taking advantage of the contained layers of air, which are poor conductors. This is the custom of lumbermen and ice-cutters, who discard overcoats while working. The chief utility of overcoats is against storms and when not much independent motion of the limbs is required.

155. Color has no influence upon animal heat, but dark colors absorb animal odors; hence undershirts should be light. All shirts should be long enough after washing to fully protect the abdomen.

156. In the field an extra shirt, for wearing next the body, should always be carried, and the two shirts may be worn alternately. At the close of the day's work the worn shirt should be taken off, dried, stretched, well beaten, and hung in the wind and sun. This should be done even when there is no change.

157. The combination of perspiration and dust is very disagreeable and hurtful, and drawers, stockings, and trousers should be treated as the shirts. The persons and underclothing of the men should be carefully inspected for cleanliness in garrison and in camp.

158. Such inspection is frequently neglected, because not provided in the drill regulations. But it is important and should properly be a part of company inspection in barracks. It should include the feet, the stockings, the shirt, and the breast. A convenient order is: *"Remove both shoes and one*

*stocking; open coat and shirt! Non-commissioned
officers are excepted!"*

159. Dirty troops are always sickly troops, and
men with clean shirts in their knapsacks at inspection
may wear soiled clothes and have dirty skins.

Breeches and Trousers.

160. Breeches are about to replace trousers, excepting for dismounted dress occasions and strictly
garrison duty, neither of which involves continuous
strain. Breeches proper extend from the waist not
below the knee, but these are prolonged to the tops
of the shoes. When trousers were substituted for
breeches in the British army about a hundred years
ago, "the increased comfort to the soldier is said to
have been remarkable." But the discarded breeches
did not cover the leg.

161. The breeches now in use are loose at the
knee, fit closely about the leg, and are tied just
above the shoe. They match the service coat in
color and material, and are for all mounted or dismounted duty out of garrison. Their fitness for
the purpose should be carefully observed, and on
occasion be reported upon.

162. Blue cloth trousers are issued for dress occasions. The cloth should be closely milled, one grade
very light, one medium, and one extra heavy, to
agree with the climate. But as their use is limited
to occasions of ceremony, these differences are less
important than formerly.

163. Military trousers and breeches should be
large over the lower pelvis, snug over the upper
hips, with a broad inner belt for secondary support.

A belt is better than suspenders, although either is issued. There should be ample pockets. Trousers used by State troops in the field should be narrow at the bottom, to stow within gaiters. Where there are no gaiters, the stockings are drawn over them in mud or dust.

164. Leggings of cotton duck or canvas are required for all duty except that of ordinary garrison or ceremony. Light canvas will wrinkle and light leather is harsh when wetted. They should reach nearly to the knee, and if well-fitted and clasped with a spring are comfortable. They are liable when too tight to lead the feet and ankles to swell. Their essential object is to protect against sand, dust, and mud.

165. Putties are long bandages running from the ankle to the knee. The British troops, mounted as well as foot, use them in Asia with great satisfaction, and they appear to be more acceptable than leggings. They are more portable and more easily cleansed.

Drawers.

166. Drawers are primarily for cleanliness, secondarily for warmth. When too heavy the soldier is tempted to discard them in hot weather, to his ultimate discomfort and occasional risk of health. They should be of three grades and many sizes and be large in the seat.

Stockings

167. Stockings are issued in woollen and cotton. Woollen stockings frequently cause free perspiration

even in the winter, when the retention of moisture chills the feet.

168. Wet feet may be uncomfortable, but are rarely harmful to a man in good health who is taking active exercise. It is when he allows himself to be chilled or to be inactive that he takes cold.

169. A wet skin or wet feet under extreme cold are dangerous. An experienced man who has broken through the ice in the bitter weather of the Northwest will not attempt to proceed until he has dried himself and his clothes, stripping if necessary to do it, regardless of the temperature, and making if possible some sort of fire.

Shoes.

170. Campaigns are won by marching, and soldiers cannot march with crippled feet. Even in the cavalry a large part of the duty is performed on foot, and shoes are potent to preserve or to damage those important members.

171. A good shoe should have a thick, wide sole to project beyond the upper leather; a low, broad heel; no seams to press upon the skin; when sewed, thread well waxed and stitches numerous; should allow one-tenth in length and more in breadth for the expansion of the foot; should be large enough across the instep, but nowhere too large nor with rough inner seams, lest the folds made in fastening chafe and the friction of the moving shoe blister.

172. A common error is an excess of leather in front of, and a deficiency over, the instep. A good marching-shoe should be high enough to embrace

the ankle, and if with a slit and a tongue in the front, like a hunting-shoe, so much the better.

173. Good shoes will last about two months in constantly marching over reasonably rough roads, and much longer under more favorable conditions. But only brass-screwed or hob-nailed soles will withstand marching in climate and soil like those of Arizona. The best heels have a narrow iron rim.

174. Campaign shoes weigh $2\frac{3}{4}$ lbs. a pair, and the extra pair required to be carried is a heavy tax for infantry to bear. The barrack shoe, or a similar water-proof shoe, might be taken for the camp; and men should be taught to cobble, which is not difficult, and to apply glued patches, and to keep their marching-shoes well oiled and water-proofed.

175. In the tropics, a light sandal for camps and garrisons would be convenient. The more nearly the foot is bare, the cooler and the more frequently washed will it be.

176. There should be a standard shoe with numerous sizes, to which the men should be confined. Few recruits are competent to judge of the suitability of a shoe, and they may easily damage their feet seriously. Unceasing and intelligent vigilance by company officers is necessary to guide them.

177. Good marching is the complement and sometimes the equivalent of good fighting; and careful inspection of the feet and instruction as to their care are necessary, especially with raw troops.

178. An infantry officer should be as solicitous as to the care of his men's feet as a cavalry officer is of his horses'. By frequent stated inspections he should make sure that the nails are well trimmed

directly across the toe, that corns or chafes are
not developing, and that the whole extremity is
clean.

179. When unaccustomed to marching, the feet
should be well soaped or greased before starting, to
prevent chafing. At the end of the march they
should be washed or wiped very clean and dry, for
which a very little water is sufficient. The feet
may be toughened by soaking in a strong tepid solution of alum when practicable.

180. A blister should be opened by a small hole at
the lowest point, allowing the fluid to drain. The
skin should not be torn. For positively sore feet
the man should promptly report sick, which will
shorten the disability and relieve the misery.

181. This powder, adopted from the Germans, is
very useful in preventing sore feet: Salicylic acid
three parts, starch ten parts, pulverized soapstone
eighty-seven parts, each by weight. It is sifted in
the shoes and stockings to keep the feet dry, to pre.
vent chafing, and to heal sore spots. It may be
more economically used as an ointment.

182. Soldiers disqualified from marching from
their own neglect should be disciplined.

Other Articles of Clothing.

183. The soldiers' overcoat, like that for officers,
is of olive-drab woollen, double-breasted, loose, extending eight or ten inches below the knees with a
detachable hood for inclement weather. The skirt
may be turned back for marching. It has no cape.
Water-proof overcoats or capes of the service color
may be worn on duty in inclement weather. The

comfort of the overcoat is still more improved in very cold climates by lining it.

184. The regulation woollen blanket is five and a half by seven feet and weighs five pounds. A soldier should not be separated from it, and in war most careful inspection is required to maintain its quality.

185. Rubber ponchoes admirably protect against rain or ground-moisture. When lying upon one on damp ground a man is spared very much risk, but he will not be protected from the subjacent cold by the water-proof alone.

186. Fatigue suits of brown cotton duck may be worn alone or over the uniform on stable or fatigue duty, or with fixed guns and emplacements. Drab leather gloves are worn with the service uniform, and white wool or Berlin at dismounted ceremonies. Both of these are for protective rather than strictly sanitary ends.

187. The special articles, such as hoods, gloves, overshoes, and overcoats of extra warmth, issued for protection against very severe weather, are fully justified by the causes leading to their introduction and the results following their use.

188. Formerly 15 per cent. of exposed garrisons were off duty several weeks each winter from frost-bite, not to speak of inability to take the field. Now frost-bite on duty in men thus protected is very rare.

189. Abdominal protectors (small aprons made of two thicknesses of flannel sewed or quilted together and worn next the skin over the bowels) materially lessen those bowel affections that depend upon abrupt changes of temperature. These are not

issued, but there is no reason why they should not be in subtropical climates, and elsewhere on occasion.

190. Abdominal protectors are not belts and do not roll up like the flannel belt. They are suspended from a tape that passes around the body and ties in front, and they lie easily in place.

191. Men should be encouraged to mend their own clothing, independently of craftsmen. A little systematic instruction in sewing would be labor well expended. Soldiers should sew as well as sailors.

192. The subject of clothes deserves careful and constant attention by officers serving with troops. Administrative officers in the central bureaus must depend in great part upon the reports of company officers as to the results reached and the deficiencies to be corrected. But such reports should be made after well-considered study, for thoughtless complaint and immature advice are worse than none.

III.

FOOD.

193. "Force manifested in the living body must be the correlative expression of force previously latent in the food eaten or the tissue formed." That is, a soldier's food must be adequate to repair the ordinary wear and tear and, if unfortunately he is yet a growing lad, to supply additional tissue.

194. Food supplies energy and animal heat, partly directly and partly by replacing expended tissue. There are five general classes of food, viz.: the albuminates (flesh); the hydrocarbons (fats); the carbohydrates (starch and sugar); the salts; and water. In one sense the air also may be called a food. These are combined in two groups, the nitrogenous and the non-nitrogenous.

195. The nitrogenous substances are necessary in the manifestations of energy. "Every structure in the body in which any form of energy is manifested, as heat, mechanical motion, chemical or electrical action, is nitrogenous." (Parkes.) The presence of nitrogen controls the absorption of oxygen from the atmosphere. "The absorption of oxygen does not determine the changes in the tissues, but the changes in the tissues determine the absorption of oxygen." (Parkes.)

196. Life is really a form of motion. It is maintained by the assimilation into the body of new particles to replace those worn out and rejected. The moment a tissue or a body is microscopically at rest, it is dead.

197. The albuminates, or albuminoids, receive their class name from their most marked ingredient —albumen. Albumen is a complex substance, chiefly remarkable for the presence of nitrogen (N) and of a little sulphur (S). Its formula is $O_{21}H_7N_{15}C_{53}S$.

198. The albuminates are found in the flesh and blood of animals, in milk as casein, in seeds, especially in legumes, and in a certain proportion in the gluten of wheat and in other cereals. The various albuminates are not identical, but are similar, and viewed as food, their value rests upon their contained N.

199. The starches and sugars are generally grouped together as carbohydrates. Starch, $C_6H_{10}O_5$, is found in all cereals, especially in wheat, oats, maize, barley, and rye; in the legumes or pulses; in rice, buckwheat, etc.; in the potato; in carrots, parsnips, and turnips. Under the action of saliva in the process of digestion, and by the aid of cookery, starch is converted into dextrine of identical chemical compositon and into grape-sugar, or glucose, $C_6H_{12}O_6H_2O$.

200. Cane-sugar, $C_{12}H_{12}O_{11}$, is also converted into grape-sugar early in the process of digestion, and in the liver it is transformed into glycogen, or animal starch, $C_5H_{10}O_5$. This is stored up in the body, to be called on as needed. The surplusage of grape-

sugar goes to make fat, and that sweets are fattening is notorious.

201. The hydrocarbons, generally known as the fats, contain much more H and C and much less O than the carbohydrates. The formula is $C_{10}H_{18}O$. The physiology of fat and of its digestion is yet very obscure, and only the rudiments of the current belief about it follow.

202. The hydrocarbons are derived from the fats and oils of commerce, but the fat stored in the body is chiefly derived from the carbohydrates. There is no present proof that fat is stored in the body as fat. Fat taken as food is broken up in fine particles in the intestines and absorbed there. It is believed that part of it is taken up in the tissues and the rest is burnt as fuel. Fat seems essential to all growth, and hence especially necessary to growing youth.

203. Fat as food is generally objectionable to the stomach in health, and its grosser forms are apt to disgust the appetite. But the wise instincts of nature allow much more of the animal fats to be eaten in cold than in warm climates. In the warmer latitudes the vegetable oils are freely consumed.

204. The main point to be remembered is that both carbohydrates (sugars and starches) and hydrocarbons (fats and oils) are necessary parts of human diet.

205. The inorganic salts are chiefly chlorides and phosphates, compounds of calcium, potassium, and sodium, not great in amount but important, and generally supplied in composition with the ordinary alimentary substances.

206. The value of common salt (NaCl) is notorious. It is found in every tissue except the enamel of the teeth, it assists digestion, and in part regulates the passage of fluids through the denser tissues. The importance of salt as a preservative of food is so great that the destruction of an enemy's salt-works is frequently as serious a blow as the demolition of a powder-depot.

207. Lime is required to make bone, and potassium to make blood and muscle, both being taken up from ordinary food.

208. The vegetable salts, the lactates, tartrates, citrates, and acetates, become carbonates in the blood, maintaining its alkalinity. These are peculiarly important, because scurvy appears in their absence. The acids from which these salts are derived exist chiefly in fresh vegetables. Their nutritive value is small, but it is a well-known principle of dietetics that they must be supplied as antiscorbutics.

209. Water is not strictly a food, inasmuch as "it undergoes no change, no chemical alteration, in the body, and hence is not susceptible of liberating force. But it contributes to chemical change by supplying a necessary condition for its occurrence in other bodies." Water makes that solution of the food which is necessary for digestion; the tissues are bathed in fluid, and our secretions and excretions in great part escape in water. It carries the solid infinitesimal tissue-making particles all through the body and bears away excrementitious matter.

210. A man dies of thirst sooner than of hunger, and the wounded require water to supply an essential

element in the escaping blood, and to maintain a sufficient bulk in the circulating fluid. Water is also of peculiar hygienic importance as one of the most common avenues for the introduction of serious disease.

211. The practical point of military dietetics to determine is, what food is necessary for the repair of waste in soldiers and how it is to be supplied. The salts, being generally found in sufficient quantities in ordinary alimentary substances, need not be considered.

212. On the fundamental principle that it is the province of food to supply energy and animal heat, the general proposition is that C and N represent the required materials, and that man needs about fifteen times as much C as N.

213. Practically the albuminates are the chief sources of the nitrogen, and the fats, starches, and sugars supply the carbon; but almost every food contains both elements. Thus starchy food does not contain starch alone, but it is chiefly starch, and the albuminates carry starches with them.

214. The problem of all diets is to secure the proper proportion of each class and form of food at a practicable cost, and to utilize it without undue strain upon the animal economy. A military diet must be sufficiently palatable for long-continued use, and be compact enough for convenient transportation.

215. Confining a man to a meat diet would require him to absorb four times as much nitrogen as necessary in order to get sufficient carbon; or a bread diet would overload him with carbon before he received enough nitrogen.

216. To supply the desirable N and C by one kind of food alone would require 6½ lbs. of flesh, or 4½ lbs. of bread, or 15 lbs. of potatoes a day, and this at the risk of disease from the surplus, supposing the whole to be digested. The albumen of flesh must therefore be supplemented by fats, starches, sugars, organic acids, salts, etc., and bread requires flesh, fat, etc.

217. All food contains water in mechanical combination, which is disregarded in calculating the nutritive value. Therefore in determining the amount of real food, allowance must be made for the contained water as about 50 per cent. additional.

218. Parkes makes this estimate of the daily water-free food necessary for a soldier:

	Garrison. Ounces.	Field. Ounces.
Albuminates (flesh)	4.31	6–7
Hydrocarbons (fats)	3.53	3 5–4.5
Carbohydrates (starches and sugars)	11.71	16–18
Salts	1.10	1.2–1.5
	20.65	26.7–31

For other tables see pars. 374–76. Besides the solids, from 3 to 5 pints of liquids are taken daily.

219. But under conditions of enforced inactivity, and especially where privation compels, life may be sustained on much less than the standard. Thus at the siege of Paris inactive persons subsisted on 1 oz. meat and 10 oz. bread per diem.

220. The ration is the established allowance of food for one person for one day, not for one meal, as many non-military people suppose. It varies with the duty of the troops, so that there are four stand-

ards, viz., garrison, field, travel, and emergency. Troops in Alaska have an additional allowance. The elasticity of the formal ration is increased by the privilege of exchanging some of its components for other articles of food. The use made of the ration by the company officer demonstrates one form of his administrative ability, as well as the degree of his interest in his men.

221. Garrison life practically corresponds to the "life of activity" of the physiologists, and that of the field is equivalent to their standard "hard labor." Where the ration is deficient, additional flour and other articles are purchased by money derived from the sale of some of the unconsumed components, such as bacon, sugar, coffee, soap, candles, and vinegar; by adding produce from the gardens, when circumstances permit their cultivation; exceptionally by the results of hunting and fishing; and by the company's share of the profits of the post bakery and the post exchange. The soldier's pay is never "stopped" for the purchase of food, and voluntary contributions are very rarely made or desired.

222. The consumption of the regulation ration in garrison is so variable owing to barter, sale, and purchase, cultivation, etc., that it is useless to attempt to judge of its fitness in one place from its suitability to another. Sugar and coffee should be saved only when the albuminates are so low as to require their transmutation into nitrogenous food.

223. The idea that the ration is in excess receives color from the excess of fats and salts in the bacon, and from the possibility of the sale of part of it when all bacon is issued. In the field, where it is most

important, the ration is least elastic and no back rations are issued.

224. The practical question at the bottom of any discussion of the ration is: Are the meat and the bread sufficient? When of good quality the beef ration is sufficient, especially when issued in such amounts that there is little relative wastage. The regulation ration of soft bread is 18 oz., and is not always sufficient for emergencies. It may be increased to 20 oz., at the option of the council of administration, by employing the bakery savings. During a part of the Civil War 22 oz. of soft bread or flour was issued, and also 30 lbs. of potatoes, to the hundred rations.

225. The present law adds 1 lb. of fresh vegetables to the ration. This may be issued as 100 per cent. fresh potatoes, or 80 per cent. fresh potatoes and 20 per cent. fresh onions, or 70 per cent. fresh potatoes and 30 per cent. canned tomatoes or other vegetables. The Subsistence Department purchases no savings of these. Unfortunately in the field, where these are most needed, questions of transportation and other difficulties sometimes limit the issue.

226. The following is a table of the authorized garrison and field rations, the latter differing from the former chiefly in being less elastic.

TABLE OF RATIONS.

		Garrison.	Field.
		Oz.	Oz.
	Fresh beef........................	20	20
or	Fresh mutton (at no greater cost).....	20	20
or	Bacon...........................	12	12
"	" , in Alaska..................	16	
or	Salt pork........................	16	
"	" " , in Alaska, when desired....	16	

		Garrison. Oz.	Field. Oz.
or	Canned meat, when fresh cannot be supplied	16	
or	Dried fish	14	
or	Pickled fish	18	
or	Canned fish	16	
or	Salt beef, in Alaska	22	
and	Flour	18	18
or	Soft bread	18	18
or	Hard bread, only when flour or soft bread cannot be used	16	
or	Corn-meal	20	
or	Hard bread	...	16
and	Baking powder (when ovens are not available)	...	.64
or	Hops (when ovens are available)	...	.02
or	Dried or compressed yeast (ovens available)	...	.04
and	Beans	2.4	2.4
or	Pease	2.4	
or	Rice	1.6	1.6
or	Hominy	1.6	
and	Potatoes (procurable locally for the field)	16	16
or	Potatoes " " " " "	12.8	12.8
and	Onions " " " " "	3.2	3.2
or	Potatoes	12.8	
and	Canned tomatoes	3.2	
or	Potatoes	11.2	
and	Other fresh (not canned) vegetables, obtained locally or transported in wholesome state	4.8	
or	Desiccated vegetables, when fresh cannot be furnished	2.4	2.4
or	Desiccated potatoes	...	1.92
and	" onions	...	.48
or	" potatoes	...	1.92
and	Canned tomatoes	...	3.2

(In Alaska, fresh vegetables 24 instead of 16 oz., and desiccated vegetables 3⅔ instead of 2⅔ oz.)

TABLE OF RATIONS—*Continued.*

	Garrison. Oz.	Field Oz.
and Dried or evaporated prunes...........	1.6	
or " " " apples...........	1.6	
or " " " peaches..........	1.6	
(When practicable, 30 per cent. to be prunes.)		
and Jam in cans........................	...	1.4
and Coffee, green......................	1.6	
or " , roasted, and ground..........	1.28	1.28
or Tea, black or green..................	.32	.32
and Sugar.............................	3.2	3.2
and Vinegar........................gill	.32	.32
or " ...."	.16	.16
and Cucumber pickles................"	.16	.16
and Salt..............................	.64	.64
and Pepper...........................	.04	.04
and Soap.............................	.64	.64
and Candles, when necessary for illumination	.24	.24
and Candles, in Alaska..................	.32	

227. When the ration was not quite as elaborate as now, medical officers of experience expressed the opinion that the flour or soft-bread component should always be 22 oz., except when on fatigue, when it should be 24 oz.; and that 4.8 oz. of flour should always be added to the hard bread. That is good advice. The bread is not quite sufficient for a hungry vigorous man. When corn-meal is issued, they thought 24 instead of 20 oz. should be the allowance. They also thought that 9.6 oz. instead of 16 oz., or 60 lbs. to the 100 rations, of potatoes, and 24 instead of .32 oz. of tea would be sufficient. All these are commended.

228. Ordinarily fresh meat is issued seven days in ten and salt meat or fish the other three. The issue of fish is a substitute for that of salt meat. When,

as sometimes happens, neither fresh meat nor the
vegetable components can be supplied, a canned
fresh-beef-and-vegetable stew, at the rate of 28½ oz.
a ration, may be issued.

229. The Subsistence Department purchases no
savings of fresh vegetables. They may sometimes
be sold to civilians and other forms of food, as eggs
or butter, purchased, but the design of the government is to encourage their actual consumption.
Unfortunately, in the field where they are most
needed, questions of transportation and other difficulties sometimes limit the issue and, issue-day having passed, back rations cannot be secured.

230. The travel ration is issued to troops when separated for short periods from cooking facilities. It
consists of

		Per hundred rations.	
	Canned corned beef............	75	lbs.
or	Corned beef hash.............	75	"
and	Soft bread.................	112½	"
or	Hard bread.................	100	"
and	Baked beans	25	"
and	Canned tomatoes.............	50	"
and	Coffee, roasted and ground.	8	"
and	Sugar......................	15	"

In lieu of coffee and sugar as such, 21 cents a day per
ration is allowed for the purchase of liquid coffee.

231. The food of troops on transports is the garrison ration, modified at discretion by the substitution
of articles of equal money value from a large variety
of other subsistence stores kept for sale on the ship.

Emergency Supplies and Concentrated Food.

232. Life and vigor can be sustained for a few
days with some loss of weight on less than the stand-

ard allowance of food. Theoretically the minimum amount is 11 oz. a day and the maximum time one week.

233. Practically, five days' full rations of hard bread, bacon, and coffee, especially if a little pea-meal is added for soup-making, and tobacco for those dependent upon it, will maintain with trifling loss of weight the health and vigor of men actively engaged for at least ten days. The half ration contains rather more of the food elements than a mere subsistence diet calls for. But the loss must be made up later.

234. The German pea sausage, formerly highly extolled, is probably overrated as a constant diet. It consists of pea-flour, fat pork, and a little salt, and is issued cooked. It readily makes soup.

235. Mixing together, cooking, and baking 1 lb. each of flour and meat, ¼ lb. suet, ½ lb. of potatoes, with a little sugar, onions, salt, pepper, and spices, makes a meat biscuit that contains about 10 per cent. water and keeps unchanged four months. (Parkes.)

236. Concentrated foods develop force, but do not supply tissue-loss, and troops operating under their spur must have sleep and the carbohydrates afterward. This is important.

237. The United States emergency ration consists of three ounce-and-a-half cakes of equal parts of pure chocolate and pure sugar, and of three four-ounce cakes of meat and wheat. These last consist of sixteen parts of specially prepared desiccated meat flour, thirty-two parts of coarse wheat-powder and one of salt, all by weight, homogeneously mixed. These, with three-fourths ounce of fine salt and one

gram of black pepper, are intended to subsist a man one day. The whole are issued in a metallic case, to be opened only by an officer's order or in emergency. The meat and bread may be eaten dry or be stirred into cold water and eaten; one cake may be dissolved in three pints of water, boiled at least five minutes, seasoned, and taken as soup; or one cake may be boiled in one pint of water five minutes to make a thick porridge. This may be eaten hot or cold, or when cold it may be sliced and fried with any available fat.

238. Pemmican, consisting of lean beef well dried, shredded, mixed with tallow, charged with currants or similar fruit or sugar, and compressed into compact cakes, contains much nutriment in moderate bulk and keeps indefinitely. It is peculiarly suited for arctic service, and is well adapted for winter expeditions in Alaska.

239. The extract of beef might make an emergency ration for special occasions, as for pickets and forced marches. It would be particularly useful after battle, and if each man could be induced to preserve a package on his person it would be of great service to the wounded. It is a heart stimulant, and removes the sense of fatigue instead of acting as a true food.

240. The medicinal use of kola certainly removes or greatly lessens the sense of fatigue and extends the limit of muscular exertion. It should not be used indiscriminately nor be depended upon indefinitely.

ARTICLES OF THE RATION.

Beef.

241. The ration of beef is estimated on the basis of the raw issue. There is a waste of 5 per cent. in cutting up the carcass. A fair proportion of bone in beef is 20 per cent. In cooking, meat shrinks about 25 per cent. in weight.

242. The issue of beef is sufficient when the quality is good, but no savings of beef are purchased by the government. Savings may be sold to civilians or exchanged. It is insufficient when taken from tough Texas cattle, or when issued in the spring from frozen carcasses slaughtered in the autumn. In cooking such meat the loss is believed to be 10 per cent. more than with fresh meat.

243. Very acceptable fresh meat has been supplied troops in the Philippines from modern refrigerating ships, especially those from Australia. This is distinct from ordinary frozen meat.

244. Beef for issue should be well grown and nourished, and cattle are best about four years old. Steers should weigh about 1000 pounds. The proportion of forequarters to hindquarters is about 8 to 7. The weight is best determined by putting average samples on the scales. Sixty per cent. of the live weight is the average net weight.

245. When weighing is impracticable, use this formula:

$$(C^2 \times .08) \times L \times 42 = W \text{ (net)}.$$

$C =$ girth behind shoulder-blades; $L =$ length from front of shoulder-blades to root of tail; 42 pounds

$=$ cubic foot of flesh; $W=$ weight. $(C=$ circ.; .08 $=.07958;$ $C^2 \times .08 =$ contents.)

Or $\qquad C^2 \times 5L \div 1.5 = W.$

If fat, divide by 1.425; if lean, by 1.575. In temperate climates beef should be killed 24–36 hours before issue; in hot climates, 8–10 hours.

246. Good beef should have about 20 per cent. bone; the fat should be firm and sufficient, but not in excess, and the flesh firm, elastic, and marbled from little veins running through it. From good meat placed on a white plate a little reddish fluid will be found to exude. This is not a bad indication, as it is sometimes thought to be.

247. The flesh of young animals is pale and moist, and that of old animals is dark. A deep purple indicates that the animal has died with the blood in it. Blood is objectionable, not because it is unhealthy in itself, but because it decomposes very rapidly.

248. None of the meat should be livid, and the interior should be the same color or a little paler than the surface. There should be no softening, nor fluid within the tissues. In commencing putrefaction the color is first paler and later greenish, and the odor disagreeable.

To Cook Meat.

Boiling.

249. For boiling, the pieces (of any meat) should be as large as possible and be plunged into boiling water to coagulate the albumen in the exterior layer, and thus retain the inner juices. After five or ten

minutes the water should be reduced to 160° F.
Above 170° the meat becomes hard and indigestible.
Albumen becomes stringy at 134° and coagulates at
160° but of course the interior of a large piece of
meat is cooler than the surface or than the water.

250. Meat is more effectually cooked at this lower
temperature than by boiling, but soldier cooks generally use excessive heat and company inspecting
officers should check them with the aid of the kitchen
thermometer.

251. Simmering and boiling are the same. The
water should not simmer, but remain at 160°–170° F.
fifteen minutes for each pound of meat. Hence so-
called boiled meat is not boiled—or should not be.

252. That actual boiling is not necessary is illustrated by the fact that meats "boiled" at Fort Logan
and at Fort Monroe are practically cooked alike,
although at the greater altitude the boiling temperature is lower.

Water boils at $\left\{\begin{array}{l} 1° \text{ F.} \\ 1° \text{ C.} \end{array}\right\}$ less for $\left\{\begin{array}{l} 600 \\ 1080 \end{array}\right\}$ feet of elevation, owing to diminished pressure.

Roasting, Baking, Frying, and Stewing.

253. The so-called roasting is baking; but meat
may be roasted by cutting it into pieces, 1–2 in. sq.,
and holding it for a few minutes before a hot fire, as
in the field. In baking, first apply an intense heat to
coagulate the outer albumen and then reduce the
temperature.

254. To fry actually is to boil in fat, which would
be excellent, but is never done because fat cannot
boil under ordinary atmospheric pressure, although

a fatty acid of butter, butyric, may do so. The appearance of boiling, the sputtering, is due to water in the lard. To fry properly the fat should appear to boil. The temperature known as "boiling hot" is shown by little jets of smoke, not steam, from the surface, and food cooked in this way should be drained for a few minutes in a sieve.

255. Slowly heated, fat evolves fatty acids, generally injurious, penetrating the particles of frying food and enveloping them in grease. The gastric fluids cannot dissolve this and it is an irritant in the stomach.

256. To stew meat, small pieces should be kept for about two hours at a moderate heat (134°+F.) in a little water. The object is to partly extract the juices, keeping the albumen semi-fluid and retaining all the surrounding liquid.

257. That very high temperatures are unnecessary in cooking meat, the Norwegian stove (as modified, Warren's Cooker) shows.

In its simplest form this is a wooden box thickly lined with felt. In the middle is a stew-pan with a felt lid. The contents are heated as desired, the pan is placed in the box, which is covered, and left to itself. In a few hours the work is done without the need of more fire. The chemist's water-bath, of which a glue-pot is the type, is an excellent cooking apparatus and in the form of a "double kettle" might well be used in all garrison kitchens.

Soup-making.

258. To make soup put uncooked meat into cold water (1 lb. lean meat to 1 qt. water), heat gradually

and cook slowly. Rapid boiling drives off the aroma and probably part of the nutritious matter. Cracked bones, whose marrow dissolves, add to its strength. Cooked meat may be added to soup three-quarters of an hour after putting on the fire; vegetables, except potatoes, one hour and a-half before it is done; potatoes, thirty minutes. The more fragments of cooked or uncooked meat and broken bones, the better. A scrupulously clean pot, slow cooking, and constant skimming are the essentials of soup-making.

259. Soup stock is made by putting lean meat in cold water, three pounds to a gallon, and cooking slowly for several hours. The fat is skimmed off and a jelly remains after cooling. This is re-dissolved by heat and re-boiling, with water and seasoning added as needed. Although rarely done, such stock can be prepared in camp and carried on the march, so as to be immediately available when camp is made again. The stock-pot should always be kept up in garrison.

Salt Beef and Salt Pork.

260. Salt beef, whose ration weight is 22 ounces, is now issued only in Alaska. Its nutritive value may be reckoned at two-thirds that of fresh beef, decreasing with age.

261. Meat is salted to preserve it, but this is at the expense of some nutritive matters that pass into the brine; so that from brine in which beef has been salted about half a pound of flesh extract to the gallon may be taken by dialysis. But brine several times used becomes poisonous, by the decomposition of the contained animal substances.

262. Both salt pork and salt beef are carried with difficulty in the field, and are not very acceptable. When cooked hard and dry they are tough and insipid Much nutritive principle passes into the brine, eaving only a fictitious nitrogenous value to the solids Nevertheless salt pork contains much more N and C than fresh pork, and is issued at 12 ounces to the ration. On the march it should be thoroughly boiled after making camp, and be set aside for use the next day.

Fresh Pork.

263. Fresh pork, never issued, is sometimes obtained through the company fund or otherwise. This and veal are liable to cause diarrhœa, especially in those not accustomed to them. Both, and especially pork, which raw is liable to carry a dangerous parasite, should be well cooked.

Bacon.

264. Bacon, containing much more N and C than fresh pork, is issued at 12 ounces to the ration. Bacon is the exception to the rule that cured meats are less digestible than fresh. Its fat is more acceptable than that of pork, it is easily transported, and is well suited to the wants of severe exercise.

265. But bacon is not acceptable to those not in rude physical health, nor to most men in hot climates, except as an occasional diet; and sometimes it wastes as much as 20–25 per cent. under natural heat. Bacon slop-fed and summer-cured wastes much more rapidly than that corn-fed and winter-cured.

266. Notwithstanding its waste under heat, properly selected bacon should generally be substituted for salt pork at southern posts. It should be stored in bins with bulk salt in alternate layers. Bacon with very deep layers of fat and thin layers of lean should only be issued at northern stations, for it can neither be cooked properly in the field nor eaten with satisfaction at the south. The weight of the sides determines the proportion of fat. Sides weighing from 25 to 50 pounds are preferable.

267. When the fat of bacon is yellow and the taste is strong, the meat is rusty or tainted; when the lean has brown or black spots, it is not good. But bacon from stag hogs or those fed on mast may be yellowish and still be good.

Corned Beef.

268. Cooked corned beef at 12 ounces is a substitutive part of the ration where cooking is impracticable. It has double the nutritive quality of the same quantity of uncooked beef, and will probably play an important part in future wars. It is issued canned. It contains 60 per cent. solids, of which 40 are albuminoids, 15 fat, and 5 salts. Nitrogen is 6 per cent. of the whole.

269. Corning is treating raw beef to a pickle, for which this is a good formula:

To 50 lbs. beef take 2 gals. water, 4 lbs. salt, 1½ lbs. brown sugar, 1½ oz. saltpetre, ½ oz. saleratus. Boil, skim, and cool gradually. When cold put the beef in the brine under a weight. It may be used in eight or ten days. This is to be boiled. After the brine has been used four times it must be boiled and skimmed. This may be repeated three times.

Diseased Meat.

270. "Bad," that is, decomposing, meat should not be eaten, but meat from animals suffering under severe and mortal diseases may be consumed without harm. While such food ordinarily should be condemned, in severe straits it is better to issue it than to allow troops to starve.

271 Animals ill and dead of the cattle-plague (rinderpest) and of epidemic pleuro-pneumonia have been eaten repeatedly without harm, and as late as 1871 horses dead of glanders were consumed in large numbers at the siege of Paris. However, it is essential that such meat be thoroughly cooked, and it is much safer that all the blood be carefully drained and not used. But tuberculous (consumptive) meat may infect the consumer, and milk from such cows is dangerous. Ordinarily, animals affected with malignant pustule should be burned, not buried.

272. Notwithstanding diseased animals are not necessarily to be condemned as food for human beings in great straits, it must be remembered that persons have occasionally been poisoned by the stronger medicines with which such animals have been treated.

273. When imperfectly cooked, beef and pork, if themselves diseased, may communicate consumption and tapeworm, and pork may infect with the trichina.

274. Tapeworm in man is generated from the measle of the hog and the ox when swallowed alive.

The measle itself (cysticercus-ci) is a small round body observable with the naked eye, and when it is numerous the flesh crackles on being cut. To speak of old and rusty pork as "measly" is not correct.

275. *Trichina spiralis* is a minute parasitic worm frequenting swine, which when swallowed by man multiplies and causes a very painful and dangerous disease. The trichinæ are killed when albumen is coagulated (160°+ F.). But if the interior of boiled or roasted pork shows the color of uncooked meat, this has not been attained. Trichinæ are also killed by hot, not common, smoking. Therefore all doubtful meat should be thoroughly cooked to insure against these three common evils, tubercle, tapeworm, trichina.

276. Sausages and pies from meat apparently wholesome may become poisonous by the formation of a yet unknown substance. Age is presumed to be one of the factors In warm weather hash prepared the night before it is to be eaten and stale mixed dishes are liable to induce colic and diarrhœa. These conditions result from bacterial fermentation.

277. Meat may be preserved for some time by heating very strongly the outside, thus coagulating the albumen in the outer layers and hermetically sealing the interior. The application of charcoal or sugar to the surface is also preservative, and gunpowder rubbed into the surface would probably have a similar effect.

Horse-flesh.

278. Horse-flesh contains more N and less C and H than beef. It is palatable and stimulating, and

horses killed in action or not required in a siege should be utilized in emergency.

Bread.

279. Bread, the other important part of the ration with meat,—for practically bread and meat make up its value,—is the only portion of it in which there is no waste. It is one of the few foods that never pall upon the appetite; nevertheless it is not a complete diet, being deficient in fat and moderately in N; hence butter or other greasy food is eaten with it by instinct.

280. In making bread there is a gain of one-third in weight over the flour used. It is possible under the concurrent authority of the council of administration and the commanding officer to increase the bread ration to the full extent of the flour ration, or to any part thereof. But if the bread is made and issued by the Subsistence Department rather than by the post or the company, the savings will accrue to it, and no increase over the authorized weight of the bread can be expected. It should be possible to change the regulation, so that even from subsistence bakeries an increased bread ration may be issued when required.

281. The weight of the bread ration is to be taken cold, because bread loses weight on standing by the evaporation of the contained water.

282. Flour is the crushed kernel of wheat with the two outer husks removed. Dough is flour mixed with salt and water. Bread is dough distended through its particles with CO_2 and cooked. Flour

contains 9–14 per cent. N, chiefly in the gluten, and
60 to 70 parts carbonaceous matter (starch, dextrin, sugar).

283. The husks or bran contain about 15 per cent.
N, 3.5 fat, and 5.7 salts. Although theoretically
nutritious, it is not so practically from its indigesti-
bility. Whole flour, so far as it truly contains the
bran, is of doubtful utility because of the mechanical
irritation. But whole flour as advertised, usually
has really little bran remaining in it.

284. "Straight" flour is the whole product of the
wheat less the refuse, with a small percentage of low
grades. A bushel of wheat (60 pounds) should yield
about 44 pounds of this flour.

285. "High patent" flour, of which "family"
flour is a type, is a very fine well-milled flour from
selected wheat and is thus of higher price, but it is
not the most nutritious. Moderately dressed or
"straight" flour is the best for issue.

286. Flour is tested by touch, color, taste, odor,
and strength or elasticity. Formerly absolute
smoothness and whiteness were signs of the best
quality; but the roller process, by which most flour
is now made, does not yield an impalpable powder
but one slightly rough, and the dark color of the
hard winter wheat ("Russian" and "Turkey") gives
that flour a marked yellow tinge.

287. Nevertheless decided grittiness or excessive
yellowness indicates, as formerly, commencing
change. Damp flour should always be rejected.
Whatever the standard, flour must be uniform in
color. Specks show imperfect milling or very low
grade. Dry roller-process flour is not as adhesive

as buhr-stone flour, but if free from dampness there may be a little cohesion on compression.

288. A disagreeable taste or musty or sour odors, indicate bad flour; and boiling water poured on a handful of flour should evolve no odor other than that of freshly ground wheat. Good flour is slightly acid to test-paper, but not to the taste. Recognizable acidity indicates change. Acid flour makes sour bread.

289. The relative strength and elasticity of the gluten make a standard for comparison between different qualities of flour, which is used by inspectors under the name of the dough test. The gluten itself is an important nutritive factor of the flour. Failure of the dough test shows weak flour from poor wheat, sprouted, damaged, or old, or imperfect milling and defective gluten. Flour from sprouted wheat makes heavy, dark bread

290. *Dough Test.*—Mix carefully flour 2 oz., water 1 oz.; when the flour is all incorporated, shape the mass into a cylinder 1¾ in. in diameter by 2¾ in. high, standing on its base; after 30 minutes it is evidence of strength if it has stood up well with a hardened dry surface; if it falls, flattens, or runs over the plate, it is a sign of weakness, of inferior milling, or of poor stock. Knead it again carefully, flatten it and pull it out gently, not suddenly, for about 5 in.; should it rebound quickly, it is evidence of strength and superior gluten. Again knead it gently, flatten it out uniformly to the size of a plate, gently and gradually pull it at the edges until it is very thin, like distended rubber; if this can be done without tearing, it shows strength and superior gluten.

291. All flour deteriorates with age, but that made from sound clean winter wheat maintains its character longest. When it begins to be impaired mites appear, and later small beetles or "weevil" are present. To purify a storehouse in which these have gained entrance, and where they will remain indefinitely, weak fumes of SO_2 must be used, although the gas will injure the exposed flour. (Munson.)

292. Flour absorbs odors readily, hence it should never be stored near vegetables, fruits, spices, tobacco, turpentine, coal-oil, etc., and the sacks should be piled about nine high, with the tiers six inches apart, in a dry room.

293. In making bread the temperature to which the dough is raised coagulates the albumen and transforms part of the starch into dextrin, and a certain amount of sugar and CO_2 is formed. It is the presence of this gas which separates the particles of flour and makes the bread light.

294. There are three ways of making bread, viz.: To generate CO_2 by adding yeast or some other ferment to the dough; to use a baking-powder, as sodium or ammonium carbonate mixed in a dry state with hydrochloric, tartaric, phosphoric, or citric acid, and incorporate it in the dough; to aerate the dough by forcing CO_2 through it. Of these the third is probably the best theoretically, because the conversion of starch into dextrin, sugar, and lactic acid is limited, but it requires special apparatus, and is rarely applicable to military service. The first may be called nature's way, but to use it requires special skill.

295. A good baking-powder for extemporaneous

preparation is: Tartaric acid, 2 oz., bicarbonate of soda and arrowroot, each 3 oz.; all well mixed and kept perfectly dry in a wide-mouthed bottle. (Yeo.) But ordinarily a commercial powder is issued when properly required.

296. The ordinary garrison method is by the use of yeast. For 20 lbs. flour take 8–12 lbs. tepid water, 4 oz. yeast, with a little potato and $1\frac{1}{2}$–2 oz. salt. The baker's skill checks the fermentation at the proper point.

297. Frequently a little alum is empirically added in making bread, its action being uncertain. Some suppose it limits excessive changes, others that it aids in the formation of CO_2. In the small quantities in which it is legitimately used it is harmless; but in excess, as in some baking-powders, it delays digestion. Alum is also added sometimes to fermenting flour so as to check the process and to enable the flour to be used, but the propriety of this is very doubtful. Within proper limits alum is believed to whiten the bread.

298. The ordinary ferment is yeast. Where this is not available leaven is substituted. Leaven is dough kept moderately warm for some time, of which a lump undergoing fermentation is kneaded into fresh flour and water so as to permeate the whole.

299. Bread is heavy from bad yeast fermenting too rapidly, or when it has not fermented enough, or when too much or too little heat is used. It is bitter from bitter yeast. It moulds rapidly from an excess of water.

300. Occasionally flour is found that is poor in

quality. Flour from sandy soil or where lime is
deficient may rise well enough, but becomes heavy
and sour as it cools. The same condition may follow the use of yeast from too old stock. Good
bread may be made with such flour by using lime-
water. And sometimes acid flour must be used,
which also requires good lime-water. This use of
lime-water corrected the deficiency in large quantities of such flour in the early days of the Civil War.

301. To prepare this lime-water, keep a barrel of
water in the bottom of which is 2 inches of quick-lime.
Stir this up well and allow it to settle in time for
each batch, and keep it well supplied with quicklime so that it may be active.

302. A bakery at the general or the secondary base
can supply a great camp or an army operating
on a line of railroad. In minor camps of any
permanence iron portable ovens will establish temporary bakeries. For marching columns bakery
wagons in which men can knead the dough, and
travelling ovens to go where guns can pass, are
practicable. For brigades or less, not in permanent
camps, the baking, as the cooking, must as a rule be
done by company.

303. The more common camp methods are by
barrel ovens, Dutch ovens, mess-pans, frying-pans,
holes in the ground.

304. The barrel oven: A barrel with its head out
is laid on its side in a hollow, it is covered throughout
with wet clay 6–8 in. and this with dry earth for 6 in.,
leaving a 3-in. opening at the top of the further end
for a flue. The staves are burned out, and for use
when heated the front and flue are closed.

305. A Dutch oven is a heavy flat iron pot with short legs and a top fitting with a flange. It is heated by coals beneath and above. It is economical to use several of them together in a trench. This is suitable for company cooking when fuel and transportation are abundant.

306. The Buzzacott field-oven and range are well adapted for baking and company cooking. The capacity of the oven is greater and its weight and cost are less than the Dutch oven, and it can be carried wherever there is moderate transportation.

307. To bake bread in mess-pans: Cut off $1\frac{1}{2}$ in. of the iron rim of one pan, leaving a rough edge; fill the cut pan two-thirds with dough and cover with a perfect pan inverted; place these in a hole 18–20 in. deep in which a fire has burned 5–6 hours and from which all the cinders but a bed 2–3 in. deep have been removed. Cover the pans with hot cinders and with earth and leave them 5–6 hours. The rough edges of the cut pan permit the escape of gases and the bread will not rise to the top.

308. To use a frying-pan: Grease it and set it over embers till the grease melts; put in dough rolled $\frac{1}{2}$ in. thick and set on the fire; shake the pan to prevent sticking; when the lower crust forms, remove the bread and set it up on edge close to the fire and turn it occasionally. One man with six pans will bake 25 lbs. of bread in less than an hour.

309. To bake bread in a hole: The simplest method is to fill a small hole in the ground with a wood fire; when the fuel is consumed, place on a stone a mixture of flour, salt, and water, cover with a tin plate and

surround with hot ashes. Regulate the heat, for above 212° will toughen.

310. To make an oven where there is a bank: Cut the face perpendicularly; make a tunnel not to exceed 5 feet in length, half as wide, and one-fourth as high; keep the entrance low and no wider than will admit a bake-pan; arch the interior; pierce it at the rear for a chimney, using if convenient a couple of lengths of stove-pipe. The chimney is the most difficult part of the undertaking. For baking, close both door and flue when heated, as with the barrel oven. Where a camp is longer than one day, such an oven may be made in flat ground by digging a pit and using one side as an artificial bank. (Munson.)

311. Bread sour from an excess of acid becomes edible when the acid is volatilized by the bread being toasted in thin slices. Stale bread cut into thick slices is freshened by being toasted, and stale loaves soaked in water and heated 250°–300° in an oven become fresh, but must be eaten within twenty-four hours.

312. For transportation loaves should be laid on their sides or ends, not on their bottoms. An army wagon will carry 1400 18-oz. rations of bread, and with side-boards 1800.

Hard Bread.

313. Hard bread is unfermented dough thoroughly baked, not burned. Bulk for bulk it is more nutritious than soft bread on account of the water being driven off, but men do not thrive on it as a continu-

ous diet. It lacks fat, which the men instinctively add when practicable.

314. Hard bread is now conveniently prepared in the form of very small rectangular crackers put up in one-pound stiff cartons, and should always be issued thus for the field. There is no waste then, as occurs with the large squares, which crumble when taken out of the original box.

Corn Meal and Oatmeal.

315. Corn meal may be substituted for flour, 20 for 18 oz., but the allowance cannot be increased, as that of flour may be. It contains as much N and four times as much fat, 6–7 per cent., and is very nutritious. It should be freshly ground from se_ lected corn, kiln-dried and well bolted. It does not keep well and, especially if not thoroughly cooked, cannot be forced on persons unaccustomed to its use.

316. Oatmeal carefully cooked is very nutritious, developing ounce for ounce 130 foot-tons of potential energy against 87.5 for bread. It keeps well, is easily cooked and, while it lacks adhesiveness for making large loaves, small flat cakes can be preserved. This is good military food. Oatmeal as a hot or cold gruel is extensively and profitably used by laborers on hard work, and is strongly recommended as an extra issue for men on guard at night or on heavy fatigue.

Cheese.

317. Cheese was formerly but is no longer issued to travelling troops, 25 lbs. to 100 rations. It is

recommended as an occasional addition to the mess-table to be obtained by purchase. Cheese is nutritious and economical, being rich in N and in fat. A half pound contains as much N as one pound of meat, and a third of a pound contains as much fat. The opinion that it is very indigestible is not well founded, if it is carefully masticated.

318. The richer cheeses decompose easily, and all are liable to do so in hot climates; hence it is not well kept in store. An obscure fermentative change sometimes develops an active gastro-intestinal poison (tyrotoxicon) in cheese that appears sound. It may be detected by pressing against it a strip of blue litmus paper, which will suddenly become red. Boiling water dissipates this poison, so that the cheese may be safely eaten after cooking.

Dried Vegetables.

319. Beans or pease (dried) at 15 lbs. to the 100 rations are part of the regular issue. Pease are chiefly used for soup, which is the only state in which men like them as a rule. It is their richness in N that makes both valuable substitutes for meat.

320. Beans contain several times as much N as bread, and supplement it admirably. But they are indigestible unless well cooked, and should be soaked in soft water about twelve hours and be boiled until they are tender, which will require two or three hours more. No amount of boiling will soften old beans. These should be soaked twenty-four hours and then be crushed and stewed.

321. Hard water is unsuitable for use with either beans or pease, as the lime salts make the legumen

insoluble. When lime-water must be used for cookng beans, a certain amount of the hardness can be removed by boiling, by which part of the lime is precipitated, and the supernatant water, if carefully poured off, can be used.

Fresh and Canned Vegetables.

322. Fresh vegetables are always desirable for variety, for their own sake as food, to give zest to the appetite, and probably as an aid to digestion and to the assimilation of other food. They have special value as antiscorbutics. In cooking vegetables there is a shrinkage of about 10 per cent., exclusive of waste.

323. Mushrooms are an agreeable addition to the company table, and when grown naturally and eaten fresh are nutritious. The spawn is easily obtained and they are readily cultivated. A mushroom should peel easily, be a clear pink, and have a curtain attached to the stalk.

324. The tomato is a better antiscorbutic than the potato. Its acid is malic, which it holds free at a little over $\frac{3}{10}$ of one per cent. and about as much in combination with bases. The tomato is excessively watery, some specimens as canned containing 97.6 per cent. fluid, but probably this could be reduced. With part of the water driven off canned tomatoes might properly be supplied, if not as an outright issue, at least at a very low price, to companies when really fresh vegetables are scarce.

Canned Foods.

325. Canned foods sometimes ferment, and the presence of gas which requires rejection is shown by

the end bulging. It was formerly supposed that
two sealing-holes in the end of the can indicated that
the gas of fermentation had been allowed to escape
through a new vent, which afterward was sealed.
But two holes are not a certain sign of bad goods,
because some companies habitually make use of two
in their original packing.

326. First-class canned goods have on the label
both the name of the factory and that of the whole-
sale house through which they are sold. Doubtful
goods have a fictitious factory name and no dealer's
name. These are easily avoided in peace, but under
the pressure of war supplies deteriorate and must be
critically watched.

327. A rosin flux as formerly used is better to
seal the cans than one of zinc chloride, which is now
more common. Zinc is charged with injuring the
health, although this has not been proved. At the
worst the rosin merely affects the taste when care-
lessly employed.

328. Canned food kept long in store especially
under either extreme of temperature may deteriorate, and should be inspected from time to time to
determine its condition. The true weight and the
nominal weight of canned goods rarely agree, and
the contents of certain trade packages are officially
estimated thus: 1-lb. can baked beans, $10\frac{1}{8}$ oz.;
3-lb. can, $34\frac{1}{2}$ oz.; $2\frac{1}{2}$-lb. can tomatoes, 2 lbs.; 3-lb.
can, $2\frac{1}{4}$ lbs.; gallon can, $6\frac{3}{4}$ lbs.

Other Foods

329. Occasionally men are fed through the company fund with a cheaper grade of food, but as a

rule (although not universally) such is apt to be defective. This is especially true of molasses, as thus bought. Speaking generally, it is not economy to buy food that costs much less than that of the same name supplied by the Subsistence Department.

330. Pemmican (par. 238) is valuable for arctic service. Pinole, or dried corn mixed with sugar or mesquit-flour, in extensive use in Mexico and on that frontier, might well be issued to scouts or native irregulars. A Mexican Indian runner will travel long distances when eating only parched corn and sugar, and sometimes a little dried beef.

331. The not thoroughly-explained craving for sugar by soldiers doing hard work in the field, demonstrated on a large scale by the British troops in South Africa and by our own men in the Philippines, should be respected. It is recognized in civil life by the extensive use of molasses on farms and in lumber-camps, and of molasses and water as a sustaining beverage in the haying-field. Cane-sugar is much more valuable than glucose, with which it is frequently adulterated.

332. Rice, the principal food of great numbers of Orientals, as seen in our markets, has had its reddish coating, which lies under the husk, removed by polishing. It has thus lost its proteids and nearly pure starch remains. When properly cooked, so that the grains lie detached, rice is very palatable; and as its starch is extremely digestible, it should be a valuable supplementary food. But boiled into a sticky paste, as is usually the case in company kitchens, it is repulsive.

333. The demand by theorists for special rations for troops, in both the high and the low latitudes, usually depends upon failure to distinguish between the food allowed and that consumed. The ration is so elastic that, with the additions made for Alaska, it is adaptable for all service. It would be unwise to impose suddenly upon white troops temporarily stationed in the tropics a diet identical with that of natives of those regions, who have become habituated to such food by the experience of generations. However their excessive use of starches, to the exclusion of flesh, probably depends upon financial as well as upon climatic considerations.

334. The bad reputation of tropical fruits largely depends upon careless selection. They should be fresh, sound, and scrupulously clean. It is in staleness, commencing decomposition, and contamination that danger lies. Salads and similar raw food from the surface of the soil are especially liable to convey bacterial or parasitic disease. Subject to these conditions, tropical fruit should be refreshing and wholesome.

335. There should, however, be a general modification of the consumed ration to correspond with this rule: In tropical countries carbohydrates form the staple; in temperate, a mixed dietary is used; in arctic, fuel foods, that is the hydrocarbons or fats.

336. Scurvy may be superinduced by mental depression and is due to the absence of the salts of vegetable acids in the food, probably reducing the alkalinity of the blood. It is checked by cheerful surroundings, and is removed by the use of fresh

vegetables, vegetable acids, or their salts. Conversely, scurvy not only disheartens the men, who lose both dash and fortitude, but its early symptoms simulate other distinct diseases. A company officer who is told that many of his men complain of "chronic rheumatism" or stiffness of the muscles, and particularly if there is a case or two of night-blindness, should look after the company mess.

337. The better antiscorbutics are lemon and lime juice; raw potato; tomato; onions; cabbage (fresh cabbage is better than sauerkraut); vinegar; yellow mustard; lamb's quarter; cactus stripped by fire (the tall varieties contain valuable juice). Raw potato sliced and covered in alternate layers with molasses is a good antiscorbutic that keeps well.

338. The best antiscorbutic is the *agave*. To prepare it cut off the leaves close to the root, cook them well in hot ashes, express the juice, and drink, raw or sweetened, 1–4 wineglassfuls three times a day. The white interior of the leaves may be eaten.

339. It is probable that the habitual use of raw or underdone flesh is antiscorbutic. Munson suggests that cooking splits up the organic acid upon which this quality depends.

Beverages.

340. Water, the natural drink of an active and healthy man, will be discussed in a subsequent chapter Coffee is a gentle nervous stimulant, and as made in garrison insures the advantage of the water being *boiled*. It is useful in winter by the warmth it supplies, and in summer it replaces perspiration. Chiccory and coffee "extracts" are harm-

less adulterations in garrison, but are worthless in
the field. In the field only coffee itself, which probably retards tissue change and certainly stimulates
the nervous system without reaction, should be re-
lied on. The disadvantage of its use in campaign,
when it must be issued ground and roasted, is its
liability to accidental loss and to damage.

341. Tea has practically the same physiological
effect as coffee. The advantage of tea is its lightness and small bulk. Its weight is but one-sixth that
of coffee. A water-proof covering is necessary for
its carriage, and the most convenient method is in
a flat glass vial. Tea is not a popular drink with
American men, and the troops generally dislike it
because of its bitterness when drawn too long, and
from the astringent taste due to the action of iron
on it.

342. The vessels for making tea should be scrupulously clean, with no exposed iron. Tea is best made
by pouring boiling water on the leaves and letting it
"draw," not boil, in a covered vessel. Should the
water be hard, it ought first to be boiled with a little
sodium carbonate. Besides having the sanitary
advantages of boiled water, tea destroys many offensive qualities of water that contains suspended and
dissolved organic matters.

The Preparation of the Ration.

343. His ability to cook the rations without waste
and to assimilate it, are marked features in the
greater efficiency of the regular over the volunteer.

344. The practical use of the ration is one of the
first lessons to be thoroughly taught, for as soon as

the stomach is not properly filled the man becomes inefficient. Line as well as medical officers are required to superintend the enlisted men's cooking (*Rev. Stat.*, 1174, 1234). This does not mean that they should minutely instruct, but that they should understand the general principles and see that they are followed. This is peculiarly important with new troops, so that a knowledge of cooking, especially of field cooking, should be sedulously taught National Guardsmen as well as Volunteers.

345. With regular troops messes of more than one company should not be allowed, because they relieve company officers of that direct responsibility for the welfare of their men and interfere with the dissemination of practical knowledge among individual soldiers. Garrison messes foster ignorance of one of the very features upon which success in the field depends.

Alcohol.

346. Alcohol, at one time part of the ration as whiskey and still sometimes suggested for use under exposure, is not desirable in health. Academically considered, taken in very small quantities it may be regarded as a food. But it is by no means the best food, and beyond very narrow limits it creates highly pernicious conditions. In moderate amounts alcohol is of immediate but very temporary assistance in doing muscular work; but the effect is so temporary, and a paralyzing action succeeds so immediately, that the work done reaches a minimum in about half an hour and fresh doses do not renew the force. The

sum total of work done with alcohol is less than that done without it.

347. The quality as well as the quantity of work done, even after moderate indulgence, is diminished; as in marksmanship, type-writing, and even in continuous marching.

348. The brain is noticeably affected by four-tenths of one part per thousand parts of body weight (0004). That is, a trifle over half a pint of wine containing 10 per cent. of alcohol will induce in a person of average weight sufficiently noticeable cerebral changes to be studied. The so-called excitement induced by alcohol is really more or less incoordination of the psychical qualities. Its anæsthetic power removes, with increasing intensity, the restraints of reason and judgment.

349. The sense of warmth felt after drinking a small quantity of alcohol is not due to an actual increase of bodily temperature, but to the dilatation of the small blood-vessels of the stomach and the skin.

350. In small quantities it exercises no influence on the temperature of a healthy adult; medium quantities lower his temperature a little, and large quantities produce a fall of several degrees for several hours.   (Binz.)

351. Its depressing effect on the temperature of the body is a cause of danger in its use in severe climates, where freezing easily overtakes those drinking; and the experience of large commands under all conditions of heat, cold, and exposure has demonstrated their greater health and efficiency when no spirits have been used.   In garrison, or with

working parties, or on forced marches, to say nothing of battle, small quantities have no influence,
and the moment an effect is felt alcohol is hurtful.

352. Its use as a medicine in disease is entirely
different from that as a beverage in health, and is a
question of therapeutics, not of hygiene. Taken
habitually, alcohol leads slowly to morbid changes,
which become permanent in all parts of the body,
and its daily "moderate" use is more dangerous
physically to the consumer than are periodical debauches. Even in moderate quantities alcohol dis-
turbs muscular action, alters the disposition, and
deranges the judgment; but the effects of similar
quantities upon different persons often are very
unlike.

353. Independently of the disease it may induce,
the untrustworthiness of the intemperate, the serious
consequences of their action and their inaction, are
sufficient reasons for discouraging the use of alcohol
in military life. And although no man expects to be
a drunkard, nor becomes one at a single step, the
entire avoidance of spirits is always safer, and to
many is easier than their moderate use.

354. Whiskey contains from 41.5 to 52.15 per
cent., brandy about 48.37, and American beer aver-
ages about 5 per cent. of alcohol, all by volume.
The inveterate beer drinker is always a nuisance,
although not so active a one as the whiskey drinker.

355. Alcoholics present a lowered resistance,
which is shown by increased liability to disease
and by a greater severity of the disease. Those
who habitually drink beer to excess are apt to have
fat in positions where it is not normally present,

the most dangerous being between the fibres of the heart.

356. The most deleterious ingredient in distilled beverages is furfural, from the more complete dis-integration of the bran. It appears to be directly poisonous, and an intoxicated person recovers much less slowly than after drinking purer spirits.

357. "The habit of taking alcoholic stimulants apart from meals is a public evil, from a sanitary, economic, and intellectual point of view." (Binz.) What is thus true of civil life is doubly so of the military service, where clear and swift judgment is required of the leaders, and prompt co-ordinate action of the subordinates.

358. Nevertheless, as beer-drinking is much less subversive of discipline than is spirit-drinking, and particularly as spirit-drinking out of garrison is a fruitful cause of disorder and leads directly to inci-dental disease, a well-regulated Exchange, wherein malt liquors may be sold under supervision, pro-motes sobriety and military efficiency by lessening the temptation to debauches beyond the lines. Although a voluntarily abstinent army would be most desirable, that is not yet attainable, and the best substitute is one content with the moderate use of beer.

359. "Vino," a crudely-distilled liquor found in the Philippines, drank in very small quantities with extreme moderation by the natives, is baneful to whites when drank, as they are apt to do, like whis-key. It frequently induces acute temporary mania, and its persistent use wrecks the cerebral centres.

360. Absinthe is a peculiarly poisonous liqueur,

which contains from 47–80 per cent. of alcohol and the aromatic principles of wormwood and other plants. Its special poison is due to these. It induces epileptic attacks as well as delirium, sometimes in succession, sometimes one alone. Unlike pure alcohol, it occasions hallucinations from the very first. It quickly and completely destroys the nervous system of the victims of the habit.

361. Wood alcohol (methylic alcohol), from the destructive distillation of wood, extensively used in the arts, is highly poisonous to drink, and the vessels containing it should be plainly marked "Poison." Fatal accidents frequently occur from the want of this precaution.

Tables of Food Values.

362. These tables of food values by Prof. W. O. Atwater, and the explanatory remarks, are extracted by permission from Billings's *National Medical Dictionary* (1890). The potential energy of food represents its ability to furnish heat and muscular or other forms of energy and is estimated in calories.

363. A calorie is the heat required to raise one kilogram of water 1° C. (or one pound of water about 4° F.); and as a foot-ton is the energy (power) required to lift one ton one foot, one calorie corresponds to 1.53 foot-tons.

364. A gram of albuminates or of carbohydrates is supposed to yield 4.1 and one of fats 9.3 calories; hence weight for weight when digested the fats have a little more than double the full value of the others.

365. PERCENTAGE OF DIGESTIBILITY OF NUTRIENTS.

Food materials.	Albuminates.	Fats.	Carbo-hydrates.
Meats and fish.	Practically all	79–92	
Eggs.	" "	96	
Milk.	88–100	93–98	?
Butter.	. . . . . .	98	
Oleomargarine.	. . . . . .	96	
Wheat bread.	81–100	?	99
Corn-meal.	89	?	97
Rice.	84	?	99
Pease.	86	?	96
Potatoes.	74	?	92
Beets.	72	?	82

—Atwater, Nat. Med. Dict.

366. STANDARDS FOR DAILY ALLOWANCE OF FOOD.

	Albumi-nates.	Fats.	Carbo-hydrates.	Total.	Potential energy.
	Grams.	Grams.	Grams.	Grams.	Calories
Child to 1½ years . .	20–36	30–45	60–90	140	765
" " 2–6 years. .	36–70	35–48	100–250	295	1420
" " 6–15 years.	70–80	37–50	250–400	443	2040
Aged man.	100	68	350	518	2475
Man at hard work, German.	145	100	450	695	3370
Active laborer,English.	156	71	568	795	3630
Hard-worked laborer, English. . .	185	71	568	824	3750
Man at moderate work, American..	125	125	450	700	3520
Man at hard work, American.	150	150	500	800	4060

1 lb. avoir. = 453.6 grams.　　　1 oz. = 28.3 grams.

—Atwater, Nat. Med. Dict.

367. NUTRIENTS AND POTENTIAL ENERGY IN ACTUAL DIETARIES.

	Albuminates.	Fats.	Carbohydrates.	Total.	Potential Energy of Nutrients.
	Grams.	Grams.	Grams.	Grams.	Calories.
Carpenter, Munich..	131	68	494	693	3194
Blacksmith, England............	176	71	667	914	4117
German peace ration	114	39	480	633	2798
German war ration..	134	58	489	681	3093
German extraordinary ration, Franco-German war. ..	157	285	331	713	4652
Factory operatives, mechanics, etc., Mass............	127	186	531	844	4428
College foot-ball team, food eaten..	181	292	557	1030	5742
Machinist, Boston. ..	182	254	617	1053	5638
Teamsters and other hard workers,Boston............	254	363	826	1443	7804
Brick-makers, Mass..	180	365	1150	1695	8848
U. S. Army ration*..	120	161	454	735	3851
U. S. Navy ration...	143	184	520	847	4998

This table represents what is eaten, rather than what is absolutely necessary.

—*Atwater, Nat. Med. Dict.*

* Exclusive of the pound of vegetables added by the Act of June 16, 1890 and of later minor modifications.

IV.

HABITATIONS.

Soil and Soil-air.

368. Soil, hygienically, is that portion of the earth's crust that may affect the health. It consists of mineral, vegetable, and sometimes animal substances, and air and usually water are contained in its interstices.

369. The air in the soil is generally rich in carbon dioxide (CO_2), and may be charged with effluvia from organic decomposition. As much as 26.3 to 54.5 volumes CO_2 per 1000 air have been found 13 feet below the surface. This air is always in motion, laterally and vertically.

370. The movement of subsoil-air is due to changes of temperature in the soil and to the effect of rain, which at first displaces the superficial and later the deeper air by changes in the ground-water. Its direction depends upon the least resistance.

371. The artificial warmth of a house draws the soil-air (ground-air) toward and into the cellar, especially when the surface is frozen or closely paved, unless the cellar is air-tight. Hence air from cesspools, broken drains, and buried decomposing matter of all kinds will pass into the cellar as in a flue.

372. Dug-outs should only be tolerated in wholesome soil, and all permanent habitations should be

88

cemented below the level of the ground or be built on arches.

Soil-moisture and Ground-water.

373. Besides air, soils contain water, divided into moisture and ground-water. The soil is moist when it contains air as well as water. Ground-water fills the interstices of the soil, so that except as its particles are separated by solid portions of soil there is a continuous sheet of water. Soil-moisture is derived in part from the rainfall, when the amount depends upon the supply and upon the ability of the soil to absorb and retain it. It is also in part derived from the changing level of the ground-water by evaporation from it and by capillary action. It may directly affect the air of habitations and their walls.

374. In relation to moisture, soils are divided into permeable and impermeable, the latter being unweathered granite, trap and metamorphic rocks, dense clay, clay slate, hard limestone, etc. However, the driest granite and marble will contain about a pint of water in each cubic yard. The permeable soils are the chalks, sands, sandstones, and vegetable soils. Of these average sandstone absorbs about 25 per cent. and ordinary vegetable mould from 60–75 per cent. of rainfall.

375. Ground-water or subsoil-water, the water-level of the engineers, is a subterranean sheet lying at different depths (from two or three to hundreds of feet) below the surface, not necessarily horizontal, in constant motion, generally toward the nearest watercourse, with changing level and varying flow, and

affected by such obstacles as the roots of trees, deep wells, and low drains.

376. Soil-moisture, the superficial dampness immediately under the surface, affects health by aiding decomposition of contained substances, by predisposing to catarrhal, rheumatic, and neuralgic affections, and by furthering consumption.

377. Ground-water by its influence upon soil-moisture may affect the health of animals as well as of men. In two stables, identical except as to the distance of the ground-water (in one $2\frac{1}{2}$ ft., in the other 5–6 ft.) from the surface, horses were constantly sick in the one and not in the other, and equal health was attained by draining the damper soil.

378. Soil is dried: (1) by deep drainage, (2) by opening the outflow or diverting the inflow. Very deep drainage is not always essential, although desirable in a damp soil. Lowering the ground-water as little as 2 feet has been known to make unhealthful sites salubrious. It is usually of advantage to substitute for a few inches of the surface soil a mixture of quicklime and ashes.

379. But newly established posts, on all but the most impermeable soils, should be underdrained 8–12 ft. deep with lines 10–20 ft. apart. In the extreme south deep underdraining should be carried out, even in apparently sandy soils.

380. Tiles once properly laid are practically indestructible. In laying them the bed should be hollowed in undisturbed soil and the workmen should excavate it by resting their feet on a berm about a foot from the bottom. A fall of 1 ft. in 100

is sufficient, and with good workmanship 6 in. is enough. With a grade less than one in a hundred, or with a bad foundation, begin at the upper end. With a greater grade begin at the outlet.

Character of Soils.

381. Granite, metamorphic, and trap rocks and impermeable clay slates are usually dry and healthful sites, although when weathered granite is said to collect vegetation and to absorb and hold moisture in the clefts. With all of these drinking-water may be limited in amount.

382. Limestone is generally dry and acceptable, but apt to be cavernous, with communicating rifts through which contaminations may pass to the drinking-water, which is hard, clear, and sparkling. In limestone ranges marshes at great elevations are not uncommon, presumably due to the retention of water and débris in the broken surfaces which characterize that formation.

383. A high ground-water and a wet and unwholesome site, although superficially dry, may be found in very elevated mountain valleys which retain the rainfall from dominating peaks (e.g., Fort Lewis, now discontinued).

384. Permeable sandstones, the air and soil being dry, are very salubrious ; but shallow sandstone underlaid by clay may be damp. Deep gravels, unless lower than the general surface, are always desirable, and gravel hillocks are the very best sites.

385. Pure sand, deep and free from organic matter, is wholesome. But sands lived upon soon become charged with refuse, the gases and liquids from

which pass through them laterally for long distances. Some sands have vegetable débris intermixed, and others have water within a few feet of the surface held by underlying clay. In southern climates shifting sands may be held by growing Bermuda grass or lupine.

386. Clay and alluvial soils generally are suspicious. Clay retains water and the air over it is usually damp. Vegetable matter and impermeable strata are liable to be intermixed in alluvials.

387. Well-cultivated soils are generally healthful, rice-fields being the exception, and these should not be tolerated near military posts, partly on account of the dampness they create, but chiefly from being breeding-places for mosquitoes.

388. Made soils, especially near towns, are frequently impure and should always be avoided for camps or cantonments. The character of the soil, much more than that popularly spoken of as "the air of a place," determines the healthfulness of the locality.

Sites Independently of Soil.

389. Unsalubrious situations independently of soils are enclosed valleys, ravines or the mouths of long ravines, ill-drained ground, in warm climates the neighborhood of marshes, especially if the wind from them carries mosquitoes to the post, and the northern slope of mountains. Through ravines there is apt to be a current of air in one direction or the other during the day and in reverse at night. The out-current where vegetation is profuse and decaying is impure, and posts should not be estab-

lished near their mouths. This may lead to marked differences in temperature and local humidity, and the out-current may carry disease-bearing insects therefrom into the open.

390. On sanitary grounds an enclosed valley is objectionable, as interfering with free ventilation on a large scale and as tending to concentrate and retain drainage. Proximity to marshes, especially on their level, is undesirable, and to be in the course of prevailing winds in southern latitudes is apt to be disastrous. In the warmer latitudes, if military posts are required near streams they should be on the windward, which in this country is usually the southern, bank.

391. In the barren regions of the southwest, camps and posts are sometimes established where there is an oasis of verdure, because it is attractive. These are generally unhealthful, on account of too high ground-water.

392. The best situation for a post is a divide or saddle-back, unless it is too much exposed or without water. Nearly as good a site is near the top of a slope, and if the crest protects against fierce winds it is better. When there is a choice, the southern is much more desirable than the northern side of mountains or high hills. But no site, whatever its altitude, unless thoroughly well drained, is sanitarily acceptable if dominated by surrounding heights.

Vegetation Near Sites.

393. As affecting sites, vegetation is classed as herbage, brushwood, and trees. Herbage, or closely-

lying grass, is always healthful. But in otherwise
arid plains a verdant oasis indicates a damp and
therefore unwholesome site. Herbage should always
be kept closely trimmed, and weeds are not to be
tolerated. All rank herbage about a permanent
post should be cut while in full growth and be
promptly burned before decay. But it is better
not to remove primitive vegetation about a merely
temporary camp, chiefly because of the additional
labor it imposes and the risk of making hollows to
retain water.

394. Belts of brush, tall shrubs, and heavy vegetation about a marsh or stagnant water check the
flight of malaria-bearing insects and form inviting
refuges for them. Such vegetation is a protection
to residents in the vicinity.

395. In hot countries the shade of vegetation cools
the ground. Evaporation from the surface is less-
ened, but that from the vegetation itself percep-
tibly lowers the temperature.

396. Vegetation that obstructs the sun's rays renders evaporation from the ground more difficult, and
the roots of trees impede the passage of water through
the soil. Forests, therefore, keep the ground cold and
moist in cold countries. Their removal makes the
extremes of temperature more marked, with an average rise. In cold countries they break cold winds,
in hot countries they cool the ground, and they may
protect against currents of insect-infected air.

397. Where they cut off sunlight and air from a
domicile and make it dark and damp, trees are doing
harm, but they should be removed only with judgment. In establishing a permanent post remove

no more trees than absolutely necessary until time
shows which can be spared.

398. Some officers dread camping in the woods,
and always select an open field. That is the result
of imperfect knowledge. The character of the forest
must be considered. The Romans habitually en-
camped under trees, and their example is generally
good. On the other hand, the air becomes stagnant,
especially in hot countries, by thick clusters of vegetation intercepting its natural currents; and in the
tropics, while shade should be preserved, the forest
should not be allowed to grow too dense around
military habitations.

399. All vegetation draws water from the ground
by capillary action, and this is afterward evaporated,
making the soil drier. An oak tree will evaporate
more than eight times the precipitation that would
occur on the area under the spread of its foliage;
the eucalyptus, which only grows in frostless climates, evaporates eleven times the rainfall; and,
according to Stockbridge, one acre of sunflowers
exhales during the growing period more than twelve
and a half millions of pounds of water. In this way
moist regions are effectively drained and made unin-
habitable for mosquitoes. Besides its efficiency in
removing water from the soil, the eucalyptus is so
repugnant to the mosquito that it affords a perfect
refuge as a bivouac.

400. Summary as to permanent sites: Avoid soil-
moisture, ground-air from decomposing organic matter, prevailing winds bearing mosquitoes, excessive
elevation, and unnecessary exposure to extremes of
temperature. Drain deeply, except through im-

permeable underlying rock; carry off storm-water; clear away brush, except about marshes; if possible cultivate grass and keep it short over adjacent ground; preserve trees, to remove with judgment later; render impermeable the ground actually built upon, and in warm climates raise houses on piers; and preserve the soil from pollution by carrying away impurities.

Barracks and Quarters.

401. Barracks, particularly if standing below higher ground, should be protected from water by trenches deeper than the foundation wall, filled with loose stone to form blind drains, from which the collected water must be led to some lower point for escape.

402. Foundation walls should be laid in mortar of cement and sand and be smooth on both faces. If not drained on the exterior, the outer space should be filled with gravel, which will conduct rain-water flowing down without the wall into the soil if porous. But if the soil be clayey or springy, the bottom of the wall must be drained, and it is better to have drains lower than the walls in all cases.

403. Cellar walls that are laid dry, or slightly pointed on the inside, have their stonework dislocated by freezing, with risk of the water passing through. Where sandstone, soft limestone, or brick is used, the outside of the wall should also be coated with melted coal-tar, and a damp-proof course be carefully introduced to check moisture rising by capillary attraction.

404. Theoretically everywhere, and certainly al-

ways in damp localities, the floors of cellars should be made proof against ascending moisture by well-puddled clay or concrete. Ordinary cement is neither gas-tight nor water-tight under moderate pressure. Where there are no cellars, the surface under the floors should also be rendered impervious, and there should be a sufficient clear space for efficient policing. These requirements are frequently omitted on account of the expense.

405. If not built of perforated brick, or made double with an air-space, house walls should be furred as well as plastered to avoid dampness. Common stone or brick is very absorbent, and, unless intercepted, moisture from rain will pass directly through, making the rooms both cold and damp. Thin walls render the interior warm in summer and cold in winter.

406. Besides healthful sites, the essential conditions of barracks are dryness, warmth, light, floor-space, and air-supply. Casemates are necessarily dark and generally are ill-ventilated and damp. That they are unfit for permanent occupation is shown by the much higher. sick-list they always present.

407. Barrack buildings must always be arranged so as to give air and light free access on all sides. That is, one building should on no account cast its shadow over another, except possibly at an end of the day, nor intercept a free supply of air.

408. Nor is there good reason for preserving the primitive and traditional hollow square in the arrangement of individual buildings. While they must be arranged with due regard to military con-

venience for assembly and drill, they should be placed with relation to sunlight and the prevailing winds so as to get the utmost advantage of locality and climate.

409. Officers' quarters should face nearly south, or should have as much of such an exposure as possible; and when two are under one roof they should not stand east and west if it can be avoided.

410. A southern exposure is warmer in winter, and on account of the prevailing winds, at least at our interior posts, is generally cooler in summer. Parkes advises the long axis of barracks to be north and south, that the sun may fall on both sides of the building. But when our simpler buildings face south, the sunlight sufficiently floods the rooms and they are swept by the southerly winds.

411. The more elaborate buildings for the larger garrisons should be planned by competent architects, not mere draughtsmen; and they, in turn, should be acquainted with the peculiarities and requirements of military occupation. Once planned, the directions should be followed throughout.

412. But however well planned, no apartment should receive more than its sanitary number of occupants which, together with the net cubic feet, should be conspicuously painted upon the door. There is a constant temptation to overcrowd, to assign a company or a half-company as such, instead of a fixed number of men, to a squad-room, forgetting that when a company's quota is increased by order the dormitory is not equally elastic.

413. In rainless regions, from sun-dried brick (adobe) may be built houses warm in winter and

cool in summer. Where the country is heavily wooded the log-house, best if square-hewn, is better than one of sawn timber, which is quite sure to be unseasoned and full of crevices. Brick, usually costly at first, is the cheapest in the end, always provided that additional quarters are built for a growing garrison and that more men are not crowded into the brick house already occupied.

414. All barracks, at home or abroad, in hot climates should be raised on piers sufficiently for free circulation of air beneath, and should have very broad verandas. In tropical regions the men should sleep well above the ground, and tropical barracks should not have flat roofs unless these are double with an ample intervening air-space.

415. The better permanent barracks are of two stories, and the squad-rooms should always be on the second floor, which is much less liable to invasion by mosquitoes. Barrack stairways should be wide, with broad steps and moderate risers.

416. Mosquito-netting is a required sanitary precaution against malaria where the *anopheles* prevails, and is still more important as against yellow fever within the habitat of the *Stegomyia fasciata*. In such regions its careful use should be enforced as a matter of routine discipline.

417. All bedding should be sunned half a day at least once a week, and blankets be aired every fine day and occasionally be beaten.

Floor-space and Ventilation.

418. In the squad-room every man should have at least 600 cubic feet air-space and 60 square feet

floor-space, and south of 36° N. these should be 800 and 70. In the tropics they should range from 1500 to 3000 cubic feet and from 75 to 150 square feet. Floor-space should be calculated according to the actual number of cots, regardless of average occupation. For air-space allowance may be made for the percentage constantly absent.

419. No squad-room should be less than 12 nor more than 14 ft. high, nor more than 24 ft. wide. Excessive width, which makes ventilation, the complete penetration of sunlight, and ordinary cleanliness more difficult, is a serious error.

420. When it is necessary to quarter troops in ordinary dwellings, the rule is:

For rooms 15 ft. wide, one man to every yard in
        length;
"   "   15–25 ft. wide, two men to every yard
        in length;
"   "   more than 25 ft. wide, three men to every
        yard in length.

421. Ventilation is securing a change of air, and the more complete with the least discomfort the better. "Perfect ventilation can be said to have been secured in an inhabited room only when any and every person in the room takes into his lungs at each respiration air of the same composition as that surrounding the building, and no part of which has recently been in his own lungs or those of his neighbors, or which consists of products of combustion generated in the building, while at the same time he feels no currents or draughts of air, and is perfectly comfortable as regards temperature, being neither too hot nor too cold." (Billings.)

422. Perfect ventilation requires a room of special construction, and thirty times as much fuel as to heat a room of the same size in the ordinary way. Good ventilation means keeping the vitiated air diluted to the standard of allowable carbonic impurity (6–7 in 10,000).

423. Air is necessary for human existence, as explained presently, and ventilation is important because after the air has been destroyed by respiration it is immaterial whether the original supply was 600 or 6000 feet.

424. Air is a mixture of 21 parts of oxygen (O) and 79 of nitrogen (N), practically $1:4$; it also carries watery vapor from $\frac{1}{200}$ to $\frac{1}{60}$ of its bulk, and it contains normally four parts of carbon dioxide (CO_2) in 10,000, and traces of argon and helium.

425. The air that enters the lungs meets in their very delicate membrane blood returning from all parts of the body, into which blood it discharges O and from which it receives CO_2, watery vapor, and perhaps volatile organic matters. This occurs by osmosis. The blood must constantly bear fresh O to the tissues or life will cease, and waste matter must be eliminated for the same reason.

426. Now CO_2 by itself is not particularly harmful, and where that gas alone is added, the air may be breathed with impunity when it contains many times the normal amount, as at certain baths where it reaches 150 parts in 10,000.

427. In a dormitory the CO_2 constantly present and inhaled interferes by that much with the release of newly formed CO_2 from the blood; and when given off by the lungs it represents that a certain

amount of O has been taken from the air by respiration. But it is chiefly as an index of other contamination that the presence of CO_2, known as the "carbonic impurity," has a sanitary value. So that the danger of living in ill-ventilated rooms is much more serious than would follow inhaling an amount of CO_2 equivalent to that expired.

428. The discomfort that persons unaccustomed thereto sustain in crowded and ill-ventilated rooms is not due to excess of CO_2, nor to bacteria, nor as a rule to dust, but to overheating and to disagreeable odors. The precise cause of the musty odor in such rooms is not known, but it is presumed to be due to volatile products from the mouth and the skin.

429. The recognized increase in disease and mortality among those living in crowded and unventilated apartments is probably due to the depraved atmosphere lessening the general vitality and weakening the germ-destroying powers in the upper air-passages.

430. Consequently, as such rooms are specially apt to accumulate germ-laden dust, their debilitated occupants are very liable to be infected with and to succumb to pneumonia and to tuberculous diseases of the lungs. And when numerous cases of tonsillitis occur in barracks, deficient ventilation may always be suspected.

431. Civilized men in their ordinary habitations may suffer from : (1) The diminution of the respirable quality of the air by the increase of CO_2 and the depressing emanations from human bodies; (2) gases, more or less poisonous, the products of combustion; (3) the compounds, sometimes odorless and sometimes giving smell, collectively

known as sewer-air; and (4) those particulate emanations, invisible and unrecognized except by their results, that cause the contagious diseases.

432. A man who loses his life by plunging into a reservoir of CO_2, as a deep well or cistern, suffers from a different condition. He is simply drowned, as he would be were fresh air excluded from his lungs by water. Possibly in such cases, however, other actively poisonous gases may sometimes be present.

433. Nevertheless besides the gradual deterioration of health there are conspicuous instances of direct poisoning by foul air combined with the deprivation of fresh air.

434. The fever of the slave-ships, the camp fever and jail fever of former times but always ready to reappear, the immigrant fever of the Irish packets of past years, and the typhus of to-day are all a similar outcome of the poisoning of man by man.

435. Conspicuous illustrations of poisoning by foul air not CO_2 are the steamship Londonderry, where 72 out of 200 died while confined in a small cabin; the Black Hole of Calcutta, where 146 were confined overnight in a space of 18 feet square, with two small windows, and only 23 were alive the next morning, most of whom died afterward of typhus fever; after Austerlitz, of 300 Austrian prisoners confined in a very small cellar 260 died "in a short time."

436. Horses transported in unventilated cars have been killed under precisely similar conditions.

437. We do not now often meet these immediately serious results of want of ventilation, but what is generally found is deficiency of nutrition, leading

first to anæmia or deficient blood, then to loss of vigor, and then to general diminution of resistance to disease.

438. In barracks the direct consequences of the presence of many human beings are always present; sewer-air and other direct poisons, except carbon monoxide (CO), are rare; and contagious diseases, except accidentally in the very first stage, are seldom found. But in hospitals the emanations from diseased bodies are constantly present and require to be neutralized or removed.

439. The problem of securing health and comfort in inhabited rooms involves preventing and disposing of dust, regulating temperature and perhaps moisture, and preventing the introduction of poisonous gases from the lighting and heating apparatus, as well as the supply of an adequate amount of fresh air.

440. A man living by himself out of doors would have so much fresh air as not to suffer from the conditions just noted; and it is the object of improved civilization to reduce these conditions within doors to the minimum.

441. Natural air contains 4 parts CO_2 to 10,000, and up to 6 or 7 parts hygienists speak of the CO_2 present as "allowable impurity." In excess of that it means too great contamination from other conditions, which is known as "crowd-poisoning." Crowd-poisoning may also occur in the open air, as when large bodies of infantry march in close order in warm weather in a stagnant atmosphere.

442. Should there be no accidental source of pure CO_2. and ordinarily there is not in barracks, all

that is in excess of 4 to 10,000 is the CO_2 of respiration, or, as it is sometimes called, "carbonic impurity." The carbonic impurity in itself is not dangerous, but it is indicative of danger.

443. The most convenient practical test for this depressing aerial poison is the sense of smell. A "close" or "musty," to say nothing of an offensive, smell means harm. To one entering from the outer air the recognition of any odor indicates 6 parts CO_2 to 10,000, including that normally present. The CO_2 is not odorous, but experience shows that these conditions coincide. A very oppressive odor means more than 12 parts CO_2 to 10,000. This is independent of the products of combustion, and refers only to animal emanations.

444. The simplest chemical determination is Smith's lime-water test. As condensed from Munson, it is conducted thus: Six clean well-stoppered bottles, ranging from 100 to 450 c.c. capacity, filled with distilled water, have the air to be examined introduced by pumping with a small bulb-syringe or by pouring out the water. From a bottle of clear fresh lime-water 15 c.c. are introduced by a pipette into the smallest bottle of air. This is then tightly closed and vigorously shaken. If turbidity occurs, there are at least 16 parts CO_2 in 10,000. If it remains clear the other bottles may be tested in succession, the occurrence of turbidity in each corresponding to this scale: 200 c.c. $= 12$, $250 = 10$, $300 = 8$, $350 = 7$, $450 = $ less than 6 per 10,000. Turbidity is recognized when a pencilled cross on a piece of paper gummed with the face against the lower part of the bottle becomes invisible through the water.

445. A man in repose breathes 18 times a minute, about two-thirds of a pint at a time. He exhales 12–16 ft. CO_2 in 24 hours, or .6 cubic foot per hour. He also discharges from his lungs and skin 25–40 oz. water, requiring 211 cubic feet per hour to maintain as vapor.

446. Arloing believes that he has secured a highly poisonous agent from human sweat, and if this is confirmed it will help to account for some of the very depressing consequences that are associated with crowds in confined spaces under high temperature, with the air saturated with aqueous vapor.

447. It is very doubtful whether disagreeable smells as such directly cause disease, but as Harrington suggests, by diminishing the appetite of those unaccustomed to them they may depress general health.

448. Air once breathed loses 5 per cent. O and gains a little more than 5 per cent. CO_2. Besides this effect of respiration much air is consumed and carbon compounds are generated by the combustion of fuel, whose products are usually conducted into the external air through flues. But carbonic oxide (carbon monoxide) (CO), one of the products of coal consumption, is an active inodorous poison which escapes freely through the joints of stoves and directly through red-hot cast iron.

449. Carbon monoxide (CO) is actively poisonous, in that it so changes the blood into which it is absorbed as to render it incapable of carrying oxygen. Because it is inodorous it is so much the more dangerous, as it is only recognized by its effects. "Less than a quarter of one per cent. by volume in the air

will cause poisoning, and but one per cent. is rapidly fatal to animal life." (Harrington.)

450. Carbon monoxide is the fatal agent in the fumes from burning charcoal, by which it is given off abundantly. It is present in ordinary illuminating-gas, and water-gas is very rich in it, so that it poisons the air when it escapes from leaking fixtures or the combustion is imperfect. From a good burner properly regulated no CO escapes, but through poor fixtures or in partial combustion much contamination occurs. Under paved streets or a frozen surface much gas escaping from the mains is liable to be drawn into cellars, and death sometimes follows. The imperfect combustion of mineral oil also liberates CO.

451. Besides the possible escape of CO, illuminating-gas while burning vitiates the air by the production of CO_2 in the same manner as human respiration. During the time it is in operation one burner, depending upon its form, consumes from 3 to 6 feet of gas per hour, and every foot burned produces half a foot of CO_2. To properly dilute it, every foot of CO_2 requires 1000 feet of fresh air. Certain other minor contaminations are also given off in this combustion. Every pound of mineral oil burned properly requires 8000 feet of air for its dilution.

452. But man is the chief source of this contamination and to keep the CO_2 down to the standard of allowable impurity requires 3000 cubic feet fresh air per occupant per hour, because a man does not breathe out of and into separate reservoirs, but contaminates the air about him which he and his neighbors must continue to use.

453. The exhaled matters do not immediately fly off uniformly into space; and diffusion, although a steady and reasonably rapid process, does not directly overcome the effects of currents caused by varying temperature.

454. When much difference in composition exists between the upper and lower strata, the upper is usually the most impure. The carbon dioxide does not sink to the bottom of the room, although probably in an undisturbed atmosphere organic particles thus gravitate.

455. For a room permanently occupied, with ordinary ventilation, a capacity of 1000 cubic feet per head is the lowest limit, but for healthy soldiers in ordinary squad-rooms in temperate climates 600 feet per man is sufficient, under proper provisions for renewal.

456. Cavalry should have somewhat greater allowance than infantry, to dissipate unavoidable stable odors.

457. Emanations from the sick in hospitals, having specific poisons of their own, require extreme dilution.

458. It is probable that the greater the amount of fresh air, especially if it contains ozone, the more rapid is the oxidation and simultaneous destruction of some disease causes.

459. Ozone is an allotropic condition of oxygen, probably arranged as O_2O. It possesses a very much higher oxidizing power than oxygen, hence when it is found it may be inferred that there is very little or no oxidizable material present.

460. All ventilation depends upon (1) the diffusion of gases, which is the property by which every

gas will freely and rapidly expand into the space occupied by another gas, practically as though that space were a vacuum, and the mixture will not separate, and (2) the entrance and exit of air from and into the outer atmosphere.

461. The diffusion of gases establishes uniform foulness as well as freshness, but has little effect over floating organic matter.

462. All natural ventilation, independently of the diffusion of gases, depends practically upon differences of temperature whereby the relative positions of parts of the atmosphere are changed.

463. External ventilation depends on heat, a conspicuous illustration being the trade winds. Where temperature is uniform over large regions, especially if it is very hot, the air may not move much and the oppressive feeling of stagnation is not imaginary.

464. But within enclosed walls provision must be made for the escape as well as the entrance of air. The simplest method is through open doors and windows on opposite sides of a room, so that the wind may blow through. This is perflation.

465. Perflation should be practised daily in every barrack, to sweep out all the air formerly present. The only exception is when rain or snow would beat in on the windward side, but even then the opposite side must be opened part of the day. It cannot be kept up in severe weather while the room is occupied, and in any weather where the external temperature is much lower than that within, the discomfort of draughts will forbid the partial opening of windows.

466. The natural ventilation of buildings depends chiefly on aspiration due, as are also the natural

winds, to differences in temperature. The outer air in motion leaves in passing over points of exit possible vacuums into which the interior air moves and thence escapes or, as popularly expressed, is drawn out.

467. The required rate of supply depends upon the size of the apartment, the occupancy being the same. Thus a space of 100 cubic feet, in order to supply an inmate with 3000 cubic feet of air an hour, must be renewed thirty times within that period, while one of 1000 feet would require renewal only thrice.

468. The floor-space should be from 60–80 ft. or more per man, according to climate and to capacity, and ordinarily all height above 12 ft. may be disregarded in arranging for ventilation.

469. The supply of 3000 ft. per hour requires the 600 ft. per man to be renewed five times within that period, and this, if the apartment is small, is sometimes difficult and at ordinary temperatures uncomfortable. Thus, through a space of 500 cubic feet supplied by an inlet of 12 square inches the movement would be at the rate of 10 ft. per second, or nearly 7 miles an hour; through 24 square inches it would be 5 feet, or 3.4 miles. In a small room disagreeable draughts would be created by such currents, but ventilation of larger spaces will be easier because in them the currents are more readily broken, although much depends on the locality and the size of the inlets.

470. But the air cannot pass out unless there is opportunity for other air to take its place. We must therefore have a difference of temperature and

an opportunity for both ingress and egress of air, as illustrated by a common stove. Hence in attempting to warm a house by a hot-air furnace, the effort "to keep the heat in" by closing the openings into the outer air fails; but when a window is raised for the escape of cold air, the warm air flows in from below to replace it.

471. The introduction and extraction of air by machinery is necessary in large and complex buildings, but not in ordinary barracks, which alone we are discussing, where the change depends upon the movement of the external atmosphere and upon difference in temperature within and without.

472. In winter, when doors and windows must be closed, the difference of temperature is a chief factor, and ventilating openings are smaller as this difference increases.

473. The following are simple methods for the admission of air, requiring no special appliances:

(1) Where the sashes do not fit accurately, wedges between them will allow a considerable current of air to enter the length of the crack and escape by the chimney or other flue.

(2) Raise the lower and lower the upper sash; air will enter where the displaced borders fail to fit closely.

(3) Raise the lower sash a few inches and fill the space beneath with a light board. Air enters where the sashes no longer join.

(4) Where the sashes are double, always have a movable pane in the outer one. But, usually, some special method of direct communication with the outer air is better.

474. For ordinary climates fair ventilation can be established by a box or tube running across the room under the ceiling, open to the outer air at each end, with a perpendicular diaphragm in the middle. The sides are perforated with numerous considerable openings, and the air will enter from the half toward which the air is blowing and will escape through the other half. If necessary the amount of entering air can be controlled by valves at the extremities.

475. Generally the section-area of inlets must equal that of outlets. Exception: Where a strong outgoing current over a large area, like a chimney, makes the indraught through small sections much more rapid. The English authorities call for 24 square inches per head for both inlet and outlet. That is excessive for this country with its greater range of temperature.

476. All air-shafts should be smooth in order to relieve friction, which greatly retards air in motion, and must be placed (1) so as to avoid direct currents between entrances and exits, and (2) to direct the air from plane surfaces, along which it has a marked tendency to adhere and roll instead of immediately diffusing itself through an enclosed space.

477. The most generally convenient method for admitting air to ordinary barracks is to carry shafts from the open air directly under the heating apparatus. Their outer ends should be turned down to prevent wind blowing directly through with violence. With a jacket about the stove, the air may be warmed before it spreads over the room; or in the same way, it should be conducted upward at the base of steam

coils, that it may not flow over the floor while yet cool. Exit shafts are to be placed in the ceiling near the eaves on both sides of the room, tall enough to use the aspirating force of the wind from either direction. In low temperatures, or wherever there is danger that cold air may enter these channels on one side of the house as well as escape on the other, valves may be arranged to prevent it.

478. A simple plan of ventilation is that of one or more tubes or shafts through the ceiling, extending higher than the ridge and divided longitudinally into two or four of smaller calibre. The air enters by one and escapes through another channel. This makes no provision for its distribution within the room, and the incoming air is liable to escape at once.

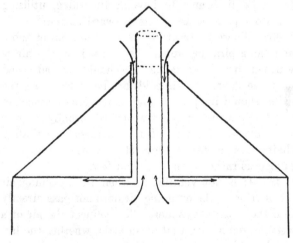

479. A better method is to enclose one tube or shaft within another of larger area and pass both from the ceiling through the ridge, the inner tube being

the longer in each direction and having flanges at its lower end. The heated air will escape by the inner tube and fresh air will enter by the outer channel and be diverted throughout the room by the lateral projections. (See figure from Parkes.) The shelf must frequently be wiped for dust.

480. Ridge ventilation, peculiarly a method for hospitals but perfectly applicable for barracks, is in substance an opening about 18 inches wide, the length of the ridge, covered by an independent roof 18–24 inches higher, with sides open in whole or in part, and communicating with the ceiling by a boxed opening extending into it.

481. In the cold season, for ridge ventilation must be substituted boxed shafts 18–24 inches square, from the tie-beams to beyond the ridge, utilizing the stove-pipe to assist the outward current.

482. Where there are both inlet and outlet tubes and no aspirating apparatus is used, if the air is warmed before entrance, it should be admitted near the floor; if it is cold, at the ceiling, and the exits should be placed reversely. Small rooms, in which doors are frequently opened, usually require only places of exit. But wherever ventilating shafts are required they should be small and numerous rather than large and few.

483. It is not ventilation when the incoming air is not fresh or the outgoing air does not pass directly into the outer atmosphere. To connect the air of a sleeping-room with that of an attic, whether the latter has windows or not, does not necessarily ventilate either.

484. Fresh air is not necessarily cold air. Air may

very properly be warmed without injury before it is breathed. No system of natural ventilation in summer will make the air in the house cooler than that outside.

485. Most walls, unless especially massive and well built, are permeable to air, and this is particularly true where the plastering is laid directly upon the brick. This permeability of walls is one reason why the apparent want of ventilation is not more serious in its results. But it cannot be depended upon to take the place of a regular system.

486. Painted or papered walls are more nearly air-tight. A hard-finished wall may be washed down with a disinfectant or otherwise when required. As a matter of routine this should be done every six months and fresh paint applied every two years. But if such a room has many occupants, there must also be numerous and sufficient openings for air.

487. The ordinary sources of contamination of contained air, besides the human body are: Leaks from sewer-pipes; up-currents from imperfect traps in waste-pipes; decomposition of vegetable matter in closets and cellars; products of combustion and leaks of gas.

488. Numbers seem to intensify the ill effects of human contamination, so "that the more men are placed together, the greater should be the air-supply per head." It is difficult to impress upon company officers the evil, as distinguished from the merely unpleasant, effects of overcrowding, for they appear lowly.

489. There is no excuse for decomposing vegetable

matter within the building, which is very hurtful, and its prevention is simply a matter of police.

490. The fresh-air supply of heating furnaces or of cold fresh-air shafts should be carefully guarded against contamination from drains and slop deposits, and the furnace proper from cracks through which the gases of combustion, especially CO, may leak into the hot-air chamber. Steam and hot-water coils do not pollute the air.

491. Ill-ventilated rooms are not immediately fatal. They cause languor, headache, loss of appetite, weakened resistance to disease, and then positive illness. For all this, increased air-space, not medicine, is the remedy. In European armies consumption, which formerly ravaged them, has almost disappeared with the increase of air-space.

492. In the French cavalry stables prior to 1836 the mortality was 180–197 per 1000 per annum. In 1862–66 it was 27.5 per 1000. In the war of 1859 10,000 horses were kept in open barracks with scarcely any sick and but one case of glanders.

Miscellaneous.

493. It is a mistake to make barracks unduly large, either in the width of the dormitory or by adding unnecessary rooms. The labor of caring for them does not compensate for the possible convenience. Wainscoted walls become frequent harbors of vermin.

494. Floors should be cleansed with the least possible water, preferably by dry scrubbing, to avoid the ultimate decay of wood and especially the lodging

and perpetuation of organic matter in the cracks and fibres.

495. On ground floors great care must be taken to prevent slops, dust, and débris generally being run under the floors and thus creating a shallow cesspool there.

496. Plaster, brick, and porous stone ultimately absorb organic poisons, which is a special liability in guard-houses and hospitals. Such walls and ceilings should be scraped at least once a year and be lime-washed twice a year with fresh lime. The plaster should be renewed at least once in ten years, and after any epidemic.

497. Steam coils in dormitories should not be placed near the walls, which means near the sleepers' heads, as is the temptation for economy of space, but along the centre of the room.

498. Kitchen waste and dish-water, full of animal and vegetable fragments prone to decomposition, should never be thrown on the ground near by, but should be carefully carried away and if possible disposed of by fire. This and all forms of exterior as well as of interior police should be very scrupulously observed, especially in tropical countries.

V.

CAMPS AND MARCHES.

Bivouacs and Camps.

499. A bivouac implies that the troops are resting in the field, with no other shelter than is carried upon the person or may be extemporized. A camp implies that the troops are sheltered by tents or other temporary structures. Where shelter-tents are carried, bivouac and temporary camp shade into each other and here are treated as identical.

500. Camps are temporary or are camps of position. The former are usually determined by immediate and imperative conditions; the latter are usually established after forethought. The same general principles of sites apply to camps as to permanent posts, and frequently both the military and the sanitary requirements can be complied with.

501. The essentials of even the most transitory resting-place for overnight are water, wood, and grass, and the avoidance of marshy ground. Wolseley advises as a military precaution always, when possible, to shield an infantry camp from the enemy by a screen of woods. This advice applies equally in barricading against the breeding-grounds of mosquitoes.

502. Men should not be allowed to sleep directly

on the ground, except in the rainless regions. A
waterproof sheet to protect from soil-dampness
should not be abandoned, and straw, hay, boards,
rails, anything but green foliage, should be insisted
upon as a resting-place. Fresh boughs may better
be used than nothing.

503. When a camp lasts longer than a day, whether
tents are used or not, the men should be encouraged
to prepare sleeping-places raised at least a few inches
above the ground. In the Spanish war, where a camp
stood in the woods, men who had been permitted to
sleep on platforms in the trees, 10 or 12 feet in the
air, retained their health, possibly on that account,
when their comrades sleeping nearer the ground
were sick.

504. In the absence of tents, protection from the
wind may be obtained within a circle of earth 18 ft.
in diameter with walls 3 ft. high. The earth should
be taken from the outside, not from within; there
may be a small fire in the centre, toward which the
men's feet should lie; the single entrance should be
to leeward.

505. Ordinarily a position on the slope of a hill is
pleasanter than one on the summit or in the valley.
But convenient proximity to water should never be
sacrificed to other advantages than that of freedom
from malaria-bearing mosquitoes. Indians and deer
rest on hill-tops in summer and in the brush of valleys in winter, and their example may safely be
followed.

506 Where trees are available, a convenient shelter is made by resting a pole on two forks, 4 or 5
feet from the ground, against which branches, thick

end up, are piled at an angle of 45° on the windward side.

507. In the field a small fire is the best for personal warmth. An Indian will squat over such a fire or lie down by it and be comfortable, while a white man builds one so large that he cannot approach it, and is cold.

508. The first duty on halting for the day is to post sentinels over the water-supply and to designate a place to attend to the calls of nature. Sinks are to be dug with the first tools. The only exception to digging sinks is when the command is very small, bivouacs after dark, is certain to march the next day, and it is known that none will follow.

509. Sinks should be placed so as not to be in the course of the prevailing winds to camp, and must be so that they cannot pollute the water either directly or by soakage. They should be well dug at the beginning, and no plea that the command will move the next day should postpone the duty, for nothing is more uncertain than future military movements. (See par. 742.)

510. The question of sinks is one of the most important and perplexing of camp hygiene. Sometimes the underlying rock, at others the ground-water, is so high that deep trenches cannot be dug. Nothing remains but to use shallow trenches, to keep regiments far apart, and to change the site frequently until formal apparatus is provided for the reception and removal of the fæcal and urinary discharges.

511. Where the site permits, sinks should be dug for each company or small battalion, but they would

better be multiplied than individual ones be too long. The most useful field-sink is a trench 2 ft. wide at the top, from 12 to 20 ft. long, and from 3 to 10 ft. deep, in proportion to the probable stay. The earth should be thrown to the rear and a layer of a few inches from it be covered in twice a day, or oftener if necessary. Shallow sinks should be completely covered in one foot from the surface, deep ones at 2 or 3 feet. All sinks should be well covered and marked on breaking camp.

512. Sinks should be screened by bushes. In temporary camps a pole serves as seat; in permanent, box seats open to the rear may be placed. In hot climates there should be some protection from the sun, and in rainy places the rain should be diverted.

513. Urinals may be placed nearer the camp, and in permanent camps it is important to have them of easy access. Some diseases may be propagated by urine, so the receptacles should be conveniently arranged and properly controlled.

514. Nothing is so demoralizing or so distinctly marks ill-disciplined troops as soil-pollution by human waste, and apart from its intrinsic nastiness it is a powerful factor in the spread of disease. Filthiness thus becomes an offence against health as well as against decency.

515. As flies may transport on their feet to the food the causes of dangerous diseases which lie in the sinks, these should be remote from the kitchens and preferably on the opposite side of the camp. (See par. 764.)

516. Flies may be diminished about a field sink by burning in it twice a day, or oftener, a little paper

or straw saturated with mineral oil. Or the petro-
leum may be poured moderately over the surface
and fired. Quicklime, when procurable, is cheap
and valuable as a disinfectant; but in some regions
it cannot be had, and its distribution in a large
army is impossible.

517. The Quartermaster's Department now supplies camps of position with a combination apparatus
which receives the discharges and disinfects them,
and at stated intervals these are pumped into an
odorless wheeled tank for removal elsewhere. As
the regulation size is only arranged with seven seats,
and as they are necessarily much more in demand
at certain periods of the day than at others, these
receptacles must be numerous in order to supply
the requirements of an army. When they can be
used they will quite replace sinks, but the more
mobile the force the less available will they be.

518. Portable earth-closets, whose contents are removed twice a day, have been issued in some of
the eastern islands.

519. The kitchen should be promptly established,
and in the same relative position as if the camp were
to persist a month. A pit should be dug near by for
strictly liquid refuse, and solid matter put in a box
or barrel for the police party to transport to a distance. When possible, a better method is to make a
deep excavation covered so as to exclude atmospheric heat, the only opening being a small trap-
door. Flies will avoid the dark interior, and putres-
cence will be delayed by the comparative coolness.

520. Old camp-grounds, always liable to be foci of
disease, should never be occupied. Only the most

vital exigency allows this general and imperative rule to be disregarded. The arrangement of a camp is prescribed by the regulations.

521. Whenever a tent is pitched it should be ditched, and as soon as the troops are rested, usually the second day, the company streets and other spaces should be marked out and protected.

Tents.

522. Four styles of tents are issued:

(1) Conical (modified Sibley): 16 ft. 5 in. in diameter at base; wall, 3 ft.; apex, 18 in. in diameter, 10 ft. from the ground; floor, 212 square ft.; air-space, 1450 ft.; allowance, 20 infantry or 17 cavalry; comfortable for half that number in a camp or slow march. It may have a stove, it has a hood open at the side and at the apex, and it is both economical and comfortable.

(2) Common ("I" or modified "A"): wall, 2 ft.; base, 8 ft. 4 in.×6 ft. 10 in.; ridge, 6 ft. 10 in. from ground, and it has a ventilator with a flap, 3×6 in., front and rear; floor, 57 square ft.; air-space, 250 ft.; allowance, 4 mounted or 6 foot men. Each infantryman would have 17 in. to lie in.

(3) Wall: 9 ft. square×3 ft. 9 in.; to ridge, 8 ft. 6 in.; floor, 81 ft.; air-space, 500 ft.; covered by a fly, or false roof, for one or two officers' use in fixed camps. In active operations officers may use tents like their men's.

(4) Shelter tent, as described later.

523. Tents are to be tan color. The conical and wall tents are for reasonably permanent camps or for slow movements in heavy order. The shelter tent is for campaign.

524. Dry canvas is permeable to air. When it is wet the organic particles are confined and the interchange of gases is checked, so that a closed wet tent speedily becomes poisonous to its occupants; and wet or dry, even allowing for probable absentees, the quarters are too close for permanent occupation.

525. Hospital tents are larger wall tents (14×15 ×4½ ft. wall, 12 ft. to ridge) that may be opened at each end and thrown together in extension. These always have flies, which protect the tent from rain and from the sun's heat.

526. It has been found that in tropical climates the interior of all tents is much hotter than the interior of ordinary houses, probably on account of the thinness of the walls.

527. Munson has therefore devised a hospital tent where the fly shall be white, to reflect the heat rays, and the tent itself drab; the fly to be 2 ft. longer and 4 ft. wider than heretofore, and to rest on a false ridge 1 ft. above the tent ridge, and 2 ft. longer in each direction; a section of canvas, 4 ft. wide and 12 ft. long, along the ridge of the tent proper, to be replaced by a rope netting. This secures adequate ventilation, and the roof opening can be closed in bad weather, in whole or in part, by a flap. In very hot weather the temperature in such a tent has averaged seven degrees less than in an ordinary hospital tent, and it has been as much as 18.5° F. less than in a conical tent.

528. Tactical considerations permitting, tents should open to the east, in order to be flooded with the early sunlight.

529. A tent is not properly pitched until it is

ditched. The tent ditch should be 6 in. wide by
4 in. deep directly at the base of the wall, and thence
follow the natural slope of the ground into the company ditch. This should never be omitted, for the
habit is a valuable one to acquire and it frequently
prevents flooding.

530. The company streets with a careful system
of drainage should be promptly arranged, certainly
not later than the second day; for very little camp
labor is more profitable.

531. Tent walls should be raised for several hours
every fair day; all the bedding and the covering of
the floor to be withdrawn and exposed to the sun,
and every particle of refuse to be removed and, if
possible, burned. In warm weather the leeward
side may be raised at night.

532. If floored, every board should be loose and
removed frequently and the ground beneath cleansed.
A fixed floor is neater in appearance, but waste matter will work through and cannot be reached. The
temptation to conceal articles under loose boards is
to be controlled by vigilant inspection.

533. Every tent should have adjacent to it an
equal area vacant, in addition to the company
street, and be changed to the new site once a week,
and the old site to be scraped and exposed to the sun.

534. Permanent camps should be as open (or
widespread) as possible, for the evils of overcrowding and the necessity for fresh air, the want of ventilation, and the accumulation of débris always increase directly with the size of the command.

535. Armies of considerable size, and especially
troops in campaign, depend on the shelter tent, each

man carrying one-half as personal equipment, so
that two men have an entire tent between them.
A shelter half is a piece of canvas 65×61 in , with a
triangular flap at one end. The halves are buttoned
over light poles, also part of the equipment, so that
the ridge is nearly 4 ft. high and the base of the tri-
angle is 5 ft. 5 in. long. One end is closed by the
flaps at an outward angle, which increases the length
12 in. Four straps let into one border serve to make
the blanket roll more compact, when the half is used
to wrap it. When dry each half weighs about two
pounds and a half.

536. In any but a most temporary camp log walls,
from a few inches to several feet high, chinked with
mud, are often raised and the tents used as roofs.
Then shifting is impracticable and the internal police
must be the more carefully enforced.

537. In camps of position in the winter soldiers
are tempted to burrow for warmth. As a rule this
is hurtful, but occasionally it may be tolerated in
very dry soil. The question should be settled in
advance after examination.

538. Where timber is available, the best camps of
position are huts. For four men Colonel Smart,
Medical Department, suggests:

Dimensions: Inside, 13×7 ft.; to eaves, 6 ft.;
to ridge, 10 ft.; door in the middle of one long side,
chimney opposite, outside of wall. On each side of
doorway a double bunk. This should be roofed
with canvas 14×12 ft. with a larger fly, both readily
detachable for transportation. This hut is large
enough, for greater size means more inmates and
relative crowding.

539. For squads of eight, the unit of the present
tactics, there should be two huts 8×11 ft., end to
end, 6 ft. apart with one continuous canvas or other
roof and doors in the adjacent ends, but not midway.
The chimney would be in the middle of one long
end. Two platforms each 6½×4½ ft., one lengthwise
and one across the end, would accommodate two
men apiece sleeping with their heads adjacent.
(See figure.)

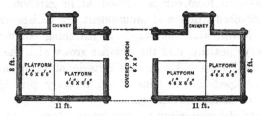

Ground-plan of two huts of four, with covered porch.

The covered porch between the huts would be
6×9 ft. in the clear, the sleeping-platform be open
beneath, and under no pretence should two-story
bunks be allowed. In the absence of timber, adobe
walls, or wattles plastered with clay, are available
for these huts.

540. Minimum spaces between huts in the same
row should equal the height of the walls, and the
passage in rear should equal the height of the ridge.
But should this encroach too much upon ample
company streets, camp must be formed in column
of divisions.

541. The intervening spaces are always to be carefully policed, for pollution there will ultimately
defile the air drawn into huts. All ordinary refuse

should be burned, if military considerations permit. Otherwise it must be removed where it will not be offensive to any camp, or be buried.

542. Hut sites and streets are to be well pounded and drained, for dry streets for company formations are important, and the whole camp-ground should be systematically freed from moisture by ditching, otherwise the ground-air will be poisoned and the streets will be muddy.

543. In fixed camps, as well as in garrison, constant occupation and amusement are indispensable for health and efficiency. A marching column is always healthy, and the sick-list grows with the age of the camp. Excursions outside of camp lines, and expeditions conducted on military principles, are of double advantage.

544. In winter camps systematic efforts to amuse the men are important. These may include dramatic and vaudeville entertainments, lectures on practical subjects by officers, and especially music. Martial music particularly appeals to most men, and good bands are good hygienic agents.

545. The dreary monotony of winter camps, the limited quarters, poor opportunities for cleanliness, indifferent artificial light, long evenings and delayed dawns, are depressing enough and lead the unstable nervous equilibrium to seek relief through the abuse of cards, tobacco, and alcohol. This must be constantly remembered, and the horrible *ennui* be dissipated, if an efficient and hopeful command is to be maintained.

Marches.

546. The direct step of 30 inches at 90 per minute for common and 120 for quick or marching time gives, without halts, 2½ and 3⅔ miles per hour. In practice it is a little more than 2 and about 3 miles respectively.

547. "The flexion step (*pas de flexion*) of the French, in which the upper part of the body is thrown forward and all the joints are bent, is said to give admirable results." (*Private letter.*)

548. Double time gives 35 inches at 180 steps per minute. It yields 175 yards a minute or nearly 6 miles an hour. This is not a marching step and is too exhausting for more than rushes and street fighting. It is simply a gymnastic exercise which should commence with very short intervals, and after prolonged practice it should never exceed 20 minutes as a maximum for picked troops. Men should be encouraged to fall out at will, for until trained up to it it is very easy to strain a heart permanently by such work.

549. The German step of 32 inches at 114 in common (3.5 miles per hour) and 120 for attack seems too long a step to be persisted in. The English quick-step is 30 inches, 120 a minute, the double is 33 inches, 175 a minute. In "stepping out" the pace is 33 inches.

550. The first stage in a long march should always be short, and with troops unseasoned in marching it should be very short, gradually increasing until the maximum is reached in a fortnight. But those

accustomed to marching drills can attain this maximum sooner.

551. One entire day, besides Sundays, in every eight or ten should be used for rest and repairs; and seasoned infantry will fairly outmarch cavalry in a prolonged journey or campaign. But if it can be avoided, infantry should not march with mounted troops.

552. Marching is influenced by the weather, the roads, the spirit of the men, the immediate object in view, and the size of the command. The ease with which troops march is inversely to the size of the command. Over good roads 14 miles in 10 hours is good marching for a large army, but a regiment easily makes the same distance in four hours.

553. If possible, move troops in columns parallel to the roads and reserve these for trains, for the great comfort of having the wagons well up when camp is made is full recompense for the somewhat greater fatigue of the route. And infantry should march with as wide a front and in as open order as possible to avoid crowd-poisoning, which may occur in stagnant air outdoors as well as in confined quarters.

554. Frequent halts are desirable: the first of 15 minutes at the end of 2 miles or less, and afterward 10 minutes per hour. At the first halt men should be encouraged to relieve themselves and to adjust loads.

555. Men should not be fretted by being held in ranks through a halt whose length is uncertain. It is no waste of time for men at every halt to spread out and rest, but they should not be allowed to

straggle. For them to lie down flat, on the face or back, is the most restful, always provided they are protected from wet soil.

556. The French save time and avoid the mud by squads of 20 or 30 forming a circle, and each man sitting on the knee of the man behind him.

557. No particular command should resume the march until its rear is well closed up and rested, and except with very small commands, leading files should not be allowed to hesitate at minor obstacles of mud and water. Jerky progression is trying to the muscles and temper of the men at the rear of the column.

558. Music is a real aid in marching; the fife and drum are exhilarant, and a full band stimulates. The tap of the drum assists a common step. Marching troops should always be encouraged to sing.

559. Raw troops invariably overload themselves at first and throw away recklessly afterward. The packs should be carefully inspected and every ounce not authorized be rigorously discarded, but afterward no necessary clothing allowed to be thrown away.

560. The authorized pack should always include a change of underwear, by preference of flannel. But necessaries should be carried at all hazards, although with new troops the enforcement of this rule is difficult.

561. Even in temperate climates new men are apt to chafe in the groins and buttocks, and they will break down with these temporary disabilities if pressed too hard at first. In the tropics such abrasions afford an inviting sphere for distressing para-

sitic diseases, notably "dhobie itch," which positively disqualify.

562. Unseasoned men with inappropriate foot-gear may become disabled from sore or blistered feet. Tenderness, the skin not being abraded, is simply bruising of unaccustomed muscles and is only to be prevented by practice walks. Soreness or chafing comes from misfitting shoes, and is usually the man's fault. The Germans treat sore feet as a military offence. All such men should be sent to sick call when the camp is reached, for relief but not to be readily excused. Permission to ride should be given sparingly for its effect on others. (See pars. 176–181.)

563. If a man who "walks on the nail" has inadvertently been enlisted, he should be taken out of the ranks at once and discharged. He is useless as a soldier. (See par. 79.)

564. Men should be required to keep the hair short, and to bathe daily the head, the feet, the armpits, and groins, the anus, and the genitals. General cleanliness is always important, but that of the groins and feet is necessary for efficient marching. The army, with any approach to equality with its adversary, that marches best will win the campaign.

565. Some experienced men when marching use merely a damp cloth on the face and neck at rising, and wash only the eyes and mouth. The face is then less irritated by the dust of the way. On reaching camp the more completely the person is bathed the better.

566. As a rule, in temperate climates, no fluid should be drunk except with meals or when the end

of the march is near.   The rare exception is for
the relief of positive exhaustion from excessive perspiration.   But canteens, filled before starting with
weak tea or water, should be carried as a precaution.

567. The sensation of thirst is in the fauces and is
relieved by carrying in the mouth a small solid like a
pebble, which creates moisture by the flow of saliva.
Abstinence from fluid while marching is an easily
acquired habit of great convenience, while the man
who begins to drink water *en route* finds himself in a
state of chronic thirst.

568. But to avoid heat-stroke in the tropics when
the blood loses much of its fluid from perspiration,
the judicious use of water to supply this waste is
necessary.   But even then the privilege is liable
to abuse, and intelligent non-commissioned officers
should be on the alert to control it.   The canteens
should never be replenished from the roadside, but
only from a regimental supply of boiled water carried along.

569. As a rule camp should not be broken before
daylight, and night marches are to be avoided.   The
broken rest outbalances any ordinary advantages
of prolonged repose later.   Except over well-defined
and open roads night-marching is difficult, and from
a military point of view such expeditions are notoriously liable to fail.   Elsewhere than on a broad
smooth road under full moonlight, double the ordinary time should be allowed for night expeditions.

570. Straggling is a serious evil indirectly affecting
the health and the morale, and directly concerning
the military vigor of the column.   All who claim to

be sick should be promptly and rigidly inspected by a medical officer, and those adjudged well be sent forward, while the ill are to be carefully transported.

571. An adequate ambulance train should constantly be on hand for the transportation of the really ill, and good troops will always repay thoughtful care by putting forth their best effort in the faith of protection when disabled.

572. A probable illustration of overmarching is the German Garde-Corps, presumably selected troops. They left the Rhine, August 3d, with 30,000 infantry; lost less than 9000 in action, and the morning after Sedan numbered 13,000 for duty; and reached Paris September 19th with 9000 present. In about seven weeks more than 11,000 men were broken down by exertion, for the camps were so short and the operations so active that little sickness occurred. Nevertheless, as a rule marching troops are healthy troops.

Carriage of Weights.

573. The soldier in the field must carry certain necessaries whose aggregate weight is considerable. It is the object in all services to reduce this to the minimum, nevertheless the British infantry carry about 50 lbs. and the continental infantry between 60 and 75 lbs. per man. It is folly to suppose, as sometimes suggested, that a soldier may have his personal belongings habitually carried for him.

574. It is the method of carrying rather than the gross weight that is oppressive. The real harm comes from the pressure across the chest and under the armpits interfering with respiration and circulation, and the want of ventilation at the back.

575. "Until some more satisfactory method of carrying the pack has been devised" the blanket-roll, an arrangement by which spare clothing and small articles are enclosed in a blanket rolled lengthwise and carried across the body from one shoulder with the ends tied together, has been authorized.

576. The blanket-roll is the natural substitute for the knapsack evolved by the exigencies of the field, but it also is oppressive in that it impedes chest movement, and it is inconvenient in affording no protection for the contents when the blanket is in use. The Parker clothing-case is a convenient refinement of the blanket-roll for the better care of the smaller articles. It is carried in the same manner.

577. The Merriam equipment, with no straps impeding respiration or circulation, with the back free from contact and the weight chiefly supported on the hips, is the most rational of these appliances, and has stood the test of experience.

VI.

SEWERS AND WASTE.

Definitions.

578. Sewage is the waste of inhabited places and sewerage the system of water-carriage that removes it. A sewer is a conduit for the removal of waste, generally meaning excrementitious waste. A drain is a channel to remove water, surface or subsoil; but house-drains sometimes mean those carrying kitchen waste or laundry water into sewers.

579. The separate system of sewerage is that which carries only sewage. The combined system carries sewage and storm-water together.

580. Sewer-air, a better term than sewer-gas, represents air contaminated with emanations from the solid contents of sewers, either in bulk or as coating the pipes.

581. A water-closet is an apparatus for the immediate removal of excrementitious waste from the place of deposit, commonly within a dwelling. A seal is a barrier, generally liquid and usually of water, intended to prevent the upward passage of sewer-air. A trap is a mechanism to retain the seal in position.

136

Sewers and Waste-pipes.

582. Sewers that carry storm-water as well as sewage should be oval in section, small end down; otherwise solid matter would lie in bars when sewage alone is passing. But separate sewers should be circular, just large enough to carry house waste and small enough to be completely flushed by it. Special ventilation must be arranged for any sewer whose outlet is liable to be closed temporarily by the tide. The combined system is inappropriate for ordinary military posts.

583. The amount of sewage should be approximately calculated in advance and the conduit built for it. Pipes that convey sewage should always be water-tight. But those intended only for storm-water are sometimes laid dry, in order also to drain the ground.

584. Small waste-pipes are the more efficient, because the friction is less, and the greater the pressure the greater the velocity with less chance of obstructive sticking.

585. Waste-pipes for single fixtures need not exceed 1½ in. and should not exceed 2 in. in diameter. For soil-pipes, 3 to 3½ in. is ample. The outlets of all waste-pipes should be full-bore, and they should join the main soil-pipe at an acute angle.

Water-closets.

586. A water-closet consists of a bowl attached to a pipe leading to the sewer. It is supplied with water to wash down the contents, and with a trap and seal in close proximity to bar the sewer-air.

587. If the water-closet bowl is not fouled above the seal, and the seal is of sufficient depth and kept intact, the house is considered safe. But ventilation and disconnection are important auxiliaries to divert the products of decomposition.

588. Mechanical closets are the "pan," the "valve," and the "plunger," all bad, the "pan" being the worst. These are relics of early styles and multitudes are still in use, but none should be introduced.

589. The "pan" closet never receives a sufficient flow of water, the pan itself and the container are continually smeared with excrement, and there is a recess,·necessarily foul, from which odorous gases enter the apartment whenever the pan is drawn back.

590. The receiver of the "valve" closet is of better shape and smaller; but it holds a greater volume of water and the valve itself is less apt to become so foul. The water is liable to escape by leakage around the valve.

591. The "plunger" is still better, but the mechanical contrivance that supports the water is liable to be smeared and to defile the atmosphere, as well as to hold foreign matter in such a way as to allow the water to escape before use.

592. The "hopper" closets, long and short, have no movable machinery, and are plain bottomless bowls set upon a trap that opens directly into or is a part of the soil-pipe, the water entering by a rim-flush from an overhead tank. The chief objection to the hoppers is that the walls may be soiled so that the natural flush will not cleanse them.

593. The short hopper is the better of the two for

use within the house, because the level of the seal is
nearer the seat and the trap is in view. For out-
houses the long hopper is preferable, because exposure of the trap to frost is less.

594. Very acceptable closets are the type known
as "wash out" and "wash down," of which the
"siphon" is an improved variety. In the two
former the bowl holds a moderate depth of water
and a deep seal lies below. The contents are swept
out by a rim-flush, which should be sufficient to
force everything through the trap.

595. One form of siphon closet acts with a jet
thrown from the front wall, and is known as the
"siphon jet." In a second, under the trade name of
Dececo, the trap is baked as part of the bowl and
both the receiver and the seal contain several inches
of water. When started by the flush the outflow
is impeded by a constriction, so that the long arm
is speedily formed and all the contents of the basin
are exhausted. The third, or Sanitas, is operated
by a column of water from the flushing-cistern held
in position by atmospheric pressure, with the end in
the water of the receiver. When the cistern discharges, the descending water escapes through the
flushing-rim and by way of the siphon.

596. Each closet should have its own flushing-
tank, to avoid contamination of the drinking supply;
the discharge from the pipe should be by a 1¼-in.
pipe at the least, to give adequate head, and the
flush should be by the rim, to scour the bowl.

597. Water-closet fixtures should be freely exposed for inspection and never be boxed in. Pipes
neatly painted should be open to the eye, or at the

most have the covers screwed, not nailed, on. Urinals under no circumstances should be allowed in dwellings. It is impossible to keep them free from ammoniacal odor, and when insufficiently flushed toxic bacteria may escape.

598. For public buildings with closets in frequent use, copious automatic flushes arranged to discharge at regular intervals are safer than those depending upon individual care at the time.

599. For troops in garrison, latrines should be in detached buildings, usually as troughs with multiple seats, and with a frequent automatic flush that may be set at different intervals if desired. They should be wide enough to avoid soiling the rear wall by diarrhœal discharges.

600. A primitive trough, whose contents escape after the removal by hand of a plug at one end, is sometimes used but is rarely satisfactory. It receives several inches of water by opening a pipe when the plug is replaced, or previously.

Traps and Seals.

601. Having secured a closet that will discharge its contents without polluting itself, the next point is to prevent the sewer-air always present in the pipes from escaping through the water-closet into the dwelling.

602. Emanations from fresh and healthful fæcal matter, however unpleasant, do not appear to be intrinsically mischievous and it is not probable that the bacterial causes of specific diseases are thus disseminated in dwellings. It does appear, however, that air charged with the putrefying products

of organic waste diminishes the power to resist illness, and that inmates of houses thus polluted succumb more easily than others to attacks of specific disease, if indeed they do not become actually predisposed to such infection.

603. The invasion of sewer-air is prevented by the trap and the seal, provided that the seal is complete and the trap itself does not become foul. The possible disadvantages of a trap are the check it may furnish to the escape of refuse through it, that it is liable to become fouled by use, and that the seal may be lost entirely.

604. The outlet of the bowl just above the trap should be a little larger than the inlet arm of the latter, the trap itself should have no recess to be fouled, when properly set it should be self-scouring, and its inner surface be perfectly smooth, which implies its construction of earthenware or enamelled iron.

605. The primitive trap, formerly in universal use and not yet entirely discarded, is the "D," which is very bad in that it always accumulates filth behind an interior recess. The more common and permissible traps, in the order of merit, are the "P" or "$\frac{1}{2}$ S," "$\frac{3}{4}$ S," and "S."

606. A running trap is a shallow U-like bend in a nearly horizontal pipe. It should not be deep enough for refuse to lodge.

607. All the water in any trap should be changed with each flush, and there should be a good supply of clean water left in the trap. This point of use is often overlooked in the kitchen and laundry sinks, the bath-tubs, and the wash-basins, so that the

water remaining in the trap is apt to be the last running out of the vessel.

608. Much of the disagreeable odor sometimes experienced about lavatory fixtures is due to the decomposition of soap and waste from the surface of the body, retained in the outflow arm of the basin, because fresh water has not been supplied to sweep it out.

609. The pipes from all the fixtures should join the soil-pipe, which is the one that receives the discharges and conducts them from the house to the sewer, by Y's and not by T's. When carried laterally such pipes should be along a decided grade, with the fewest possible changes of direction. Water-closets should join the soil-pipe at an acute angle, and over as short a route as possible.

610. A seal may be forced by the sheer momentum of the water pouring through it, it may evaporate, it may be broken by back-pressure or by siphonage

611. Serious evaporation is not likely to occur where a closet is in use. But where a fixture is not in use, as when the house or a part of it is closed, the trap should be filled with a heavy oil or with glycerine. Leakage by the capillary action of threads, hair, etc., caught in the trap, sometimes carries off the seal.

612. Back-pressure is the consequence of a heavy column of water descending the main soil-pipe to near its end, where there is an abrupt bend or some other obstacle to the escape of the air in front of it This air being compressed, moves in the direction of the least resistance up the nearest branch pipe and through the seal. To produce back-pressure the

descending column must have acquired considerable velocity, and there must be an impediment to the escape of the air before it. The fixture whose trap is forced will therefore be near the bottom of the stack.

613. Siphonage is the effect of a heavy column of water falling suddenly down a soil-pipe and thus producing a partial vacuum, by which the equilibrium of the seal is destroyed and it is broken by atmospheric pressure from within the closet. It is most apt to occur to the highest seal in a tall stack.

614. Back-pressure and siphonage are complemental, and both cannot occur to the same fixture.

615. A vent is a pipe in the upper bend of the trap connecting with either the soil-pipe or a general vent-pipe, to admit air and so prevent siphonage. It will also counteract back-pressure. It is chiefly required in large houses or those with complicated systems of plumbing. Its best location is on the soil-pipe just beyond the crown of the trap. If it joins a general vent-pipe, it should be at a point higher than the level of the water in the fixture. The vent should be the full size of the trap, at least up to two inches. Venting waste-pipes and ventilating soil-pipes are distinct.

616. The objections to vents are their liability to become clogged by undissolved matters splashing against the opening in the trap, and their tendency to evaporate the seal.

617. A trap-vent that preserves the equilibrium by introducing fresh air from the interior of the dwelling, and uses mercury to prevent the backward flow, is widely used and appears to be satisfactory

618. There are other difficulties to be met with in plumbing, and it is not sufficient for a quartermaster to assume that because a contract has been made to introduce fixtures that that is all that is necessary; nor for a commanding officer to suppose that if, when plumbing is complained of, no broken pipe nor leaking joint can be found, nothing is amiss.

The Soil-pipe.

619. The soil-pipe should be of iron within the house and of earthenware (tile) outside of it. Leaden pipes, formerly used, are liable to corrosion and to be gnawed by rats. Outside of the house it is sometimes called the branch sewer-pipe, and sometimes, but improperly, the house-drain. Where it passes out of the house it should be protected by an arch in the wall.

620. It should have a calibre not to exceed 4 inches for large public buildings, while from 3 to 3½ inches is ample for 'ordinary private houses. It must extend full-bore above the roof and in cold climates be somewhat larger at the exit, on account of accumulating frost, and the end should not be curved nor be covered by a cowl.

621. The soil-pipe should have few changes of d.rection and those over as large curves as possible, and should never be carried horizontally nor under buildings if it can be avoided. The part above the upper closet must be of the same material and construction as the remainder, to prevent leaking of gases.

622. The part above the roof should terminate below the level of the chimney-top, and not be near

a window into which the gases from it may drift. Neither the soil-pipe nor the vent-pipe should be allowed to terminate within a chimney, as is sometimes done, because the fires are not perpetual and down drafts frequently occur. Such pipes also are liable to be choked with soot.

623. In large houses the vent-pipes are sometimes run together upward in a single pipe. In smaller houses they may enter the soil-pipe above the highest fixture. That is usually quite sufficient.

624. The entire soil-pipe should be tested for leaks by water pressure when set up. Afterward suspected leaks are searched for by peppermint or smoke.

Disconnection.

625. A sewer is "disconnected" when there is a large vent, either with or without a running-trap, outside of the house, allowing the free ingress of fresh air or the exit of foul air, as the pressure may determine. The "disconnection" is conventional rather than actual, and it is difficult to carry out in snowy or very cold climates.

626. The running-trap may be dispensed with when the sewer into which the soil-pipe discharges is fairly kept, or if it is liable to be frozen, or if the grade is not good. It is chiefly required in houses not connected with a good sewer system. When this trap is used, there must be a vent between it and the house.

Ventilation of Sewers.

627. The third and very important method of preventing house infection from sewers is by ventilation,

which means the free passage of air through the soil-pipe, thus relieving the seal of undue pressure. This is accomplished by extending the soil-pipe full calibre above the highest closet and through the roof into the open air, with the top free and with no obstacle from end to end except, possibly, the running-trap.

628. But as ventilation requires an inlet as well as an outlet, there should be a disconnecting vent of full size in the pipe line between the house and the sewer. Generally speaking, sewer-air will not escape by this vent, but will rise in the heated soil-pipe within the house; nevertheless, windows or air-ducts into the house should not be near the vent.

629. Rain leaders sometimes conduct storm-water from the roofs into the sewers. They will ventilate upward as well as carry water down, and therefore those near windows should not be thus used. Under no circumstances should they discharge on the sewer side of the trap or of the vent, and there always should be a vent.

630. It occasionally happens that, impressed with the desirability of removing sewage from habitations, post authorities have used wooden drains through which to discharge such excreta. It is only a short time before such conduits become clogged and saturated with their contents, and are thus transformed into long permanent cesspools. If used at all, they must be set so that one angle forms the lowest line.

Privies, etc.

631. But water-carriage of excreta is the exception in the army; nevertheless excreta and garbage generally must be disposed of, and that promptly. At posts after a well-ordered sewer system come, in order of desirability, (1) closets over the water, as may be arranged on the seacoast; (2) cesspools; (3) privies; (4) the dry-earth system, and, chiefly for the future, the furnace for the disposal of garbage.

632. A cesspool is a cistern, generally walled dry, with a floor of earth. Into this the house waste is conducted by pipes, and from it the liquid matters drain and the solids are removed as required. For its proper use the soil must be porous, the groundwater low, and the water-supply be beyond reach of contamination.

633. A deep dry-walled privy, covered and when full abandoned, is a variety common at some posts. These should be, but rarely are, permanently marked to warn future garrisons.

634. The worst privies are the common shallow pits dug for temporary relief, generally without authority, near stables, corrals, and married men's quarters. These are often filled to repletion, insufficiently covered and unmarked, honeycombing an old post. They should only be dug by authority specifically designating place and depth, be filled in according to rule when no longer to be used, and marked in place and on the post map. Such care is especially important when the water is drawn from wells or superficial reservoirs.

635. The dry-earth system depends for its efficacy

on the deodorizing power of really dry earth or ashes covering the discharges at once. This is extremely difficult to carry out systematically and well, especially under the conditions of garrison life.

636. Sometimes the discharges are transported in movable drawers at daily intervals to another place of deposit, but always with considerable risk of distributing part of their contents.

637. All human excreta should be carefully disposed of by burial or by fire. It is not sufficient that they are out of sight. The disinfection and disposition of hospital refuse is a distinct subject, for the Medical Department to carry out.

Kitchen Slops.

638. Kitchen and laundry slops are liable to be hurtful, because they contain in solution and suspension animal and vegetable débris, which certainly undergo decomposition and are liable to be charged with emanations from the body in disease as well as in health. The ground on which slops are habitually thrown is often indescribably foul by soakage, and yet few people suspect such waste to be harmful.

639. All waste going out of a house, not into sewers, should be received in water-tight barrels, which should rest on platforms that are movable, or so arranged that the ground under them can be cleaned.

640. The ultimate destruction of all garbage is best accomplished by fire. Garbage furnaces that effectually destroy all refuse without odor and at moderate cost are now in use in many cities and at some posts.

641. Pending that, and in the absence of deep water, refuse should be carefully separated into the destructible (organic débris), like slops, old clothes, decaying vegetables, and the indestructible, as tin cans, pottery, etc. The former should be buried in deep and remote trenches when the weather permits, and the latter be cast away by itself.

642. When water is introduced into a post by a pipe system, pains must be taken at the same time to have it systematically carried away; otherwise the surplus water will saturate the ground, often already full of organic waste, and under heat disease will arise. This oversight occasionally occurs.

VII.

WATER.

Sources.

643. Water, which is more immediately necessary to life than is food, has its ultimate general source in the clouds, which are replenished by evaporation. But most drinking-water is directly derived from streams (including ponds), springs, or wells. The rain which soaks directly into the ground, either at hand or afar, and is held by an impenetrable stratum, constitutes subsoil water.

644. But a deep water-supply is almost everywhere to be found below the subsoil or ground-water. This is derived from rain-water following the lines of upturned strata directly through impervious layers, until it is held at a great depth either in local reservoirs or in immense beds whose origin may be far distant.

645. Water that appears on the surface in limited quantities is called a spring. This may have a strictly local origin and temporary life, being derived from a rainfall upon a neighboring hill; or it may be a permanent flow, the manifestation of a deep-seated supply from a very distant source.

Cisterns.

646. Rain-water, collected from a clean surface, after the atmosphere has been well washed, is the purest in nature; but its storage is so difficult as to degrade cistern-water from the first rank.

647. In collecting cistern-water, unless the surface is very clean, the first rainfall should run to waste or be very carefully filtered, for the washings of roofs introduce a rapidly-decomposing sediment. Dust should be washed out of the air charged with it, before the rainfall is secured.

648. Cisterns rapidly deteriorate, and when of wood the fluctuating water-line fosters decay. But clean gravel will introduce into wooden cisterns the bacteria of nitrification, which are purifying agents. Underground cisterns, usually of cement-lined brick, are liable to leakage into them through cracks or from the surface. Overflow-pipes of cisterns should not connect with sewers lest foul air come over and be absorbed.

649. The quantity of water that may be collected from a non-absorbent surface is determined by multiplying the area by the rainfall. Thus: Reduce square feet to inches ($\times 144$), and multiply this by inches of rain, which will equal cubic inches of rain. Divide this by 1728 for cubic feet, or by 277.274 for gallons. The area of roofs is that of the horizontal plane covered, not of the slopes.

Springs and Wells.

650. Springs whose origin is remote from habitations, large lakes, and streams flowing through unin-

habited regions furnish the best sources of water-supply, except rain-water from a perfectly clean surface in a protected reservoir.

651. Wells may obtain their water from either the ground-water or the deep supply, and it is practically impossible to determine from which without a fair knowledge of the local geology.

652. The arbitrary rule, to which there are many exceptions, is: Wells less than 50 feet deep are shallow, from subsoil water; more than 50 feet deep, from deep water-bearing levels.

653. Neither does the depth of the well determine off-hand the source of the water. For example: London and Paris both lie over impervious basins into which water drains from great distances, and can be reached by the artesian method. But New York is underlaid by rocks lying nearly perpendicular to the horizon, so that its subjacent water is practically surface water that has soaked directly downward.

654. If the surface is not polluted, water in shallow wells is as good as that in deep wells. But where the soil is contaminated it is only a question of time when the well, whatever its depth, whose water passes through it, becomes equally foul with a shallow one. The longer and the more densely the neighborhood has been inhabited, the greater the risk. Ordinary well-water in an inhabited region is doubtful, and houses standing 100 feet apart should condemn all intervening wells.

655. The rule is general that wells drain inverted cones whose radius equals their depth. In sand the area is much greater; and any well may receive a supply, pure or impure, through a fault.

656. The most of the water in a well on the bank of a river does not come from the river, but from the intercepted subsoil water making its way toward the stream. Speaking generally, the silt lining the river-bed makes a coating impervious to the outward flow of water.

657. Wells should collect ground-water going toward, not coming from, a polluted site; and no well, even in search of deep water, should pierce a polluted basin, because the shaft is liable to conduct water from the upper to the lower level.

658. When necessary, water can usually be found in the dry bed of a "sunk" river; or good water may be obtained by piercing the bed of a polluted stream and pumping through a water-tight casing from the parallel subfluvial flow.

659. Water found by the sea is usually brackish, but if a large underground volume of fresh water flows from higher ground it may hold back the salt water, so that wells very near the shore may be fresh. When brackish water is found, if wells are sunk inland in succession the influence of the salt may finally be avoided. (Parkes.)

660. In searching for water, Parkes advises that, on a plain, depressions in the surface should be tested; that even on a sandy plain morning mists or swarms of insects indicate water comparatively near the surface, and that where there is most herbage water is more likely to be found. (See par. 391.) He also advises among hills to sink wells at the lowest point, not on a spur; at the junction of valleys; and always on the side of a valley next to the higher ground.

Solution and Suspension.

661. Outside of the laboratory there is no perfectly pure water, as by its very great solvent power
it takes up portions of innumerable substances that
come in contact with it; besides which it holds in
suspension many undissolved foreign bodies accidentally introduced.

662. Water may contain mineral matter in solution, mineral and organic matters in suspension, and
organic matter in solution of varying qualities, some
harmless and some accompanied by, if not distinctly made up of, specific disease-causes.

663. Substances in solution completely disappear
and cannot be filtered out; e.g., salt or sugar. In
suspension the particles do not entirely disappear,
and their presence is shown by turbidity or opacity.
Nevertheless, water may be colored and at least
translucent; e.g., solution of sulphate of copper,
cypress-swamp water.

664. Dissolved matter can only be removed by
chemical action, or by reducing through evaporation
(distillation) the proportion of water so that a part
of the contained solid is precipitated.

665. The alkaline waters of the plains carry great
quantities of soda, potash, or magnesia, and are conspicuous examples on a large scale of watery solu-
tions. As far as known, they may only be purified
by distillation. They are more disagreeable in the
rainy season, because the alkali left on the surface of
the soil by evaporation in the dry weather is then
washed into the wells.

Hard Water.

666. Water is arbitrarily regarded as hard or soft, as it contains more or less than ten grains of mineral matter to the gallon. Practically that "which flows through calcareous channels is hard, and that which flows through silicious rocks is soft."

667. The hardness of water is caused by the presence of lime, magnesia, iron, baryta, alumina, or certain other minerals. It renders cooking of certain vegetables very difficult and compels the use of a great deal of extra soap to neutralize it before washing can be done. It is thus of economical importance.

668. Hard water is generally bright and sparkling. Persons accustomed to drinking soft water generally have some intestinal trouble after drinking hard water, and the reverse is true. But other sanitary conditions being equal, mortality is not influenced by the hardness or softness of the water-supply.

669. In practice hardness is recognized by the curdling that follows when there is an attempt to dissolve soap in the water. Soaps are alkaline oleates which quickly form a lather when mixed with pure water. But if the substances that give hardness to the water are present, oleates of those bases are formed and no lather is given until the bases are thrown down.

670. Resting upon the foregoing is the soap test for hardness, where a standard solution of soap is used to neutralize these bases, and the degrees are established according to a certain scale.

To Remove the Hardness of Water.

671. The hardness of water is divided into temporary and permanent or fixed, the sum of the two constituting the total hardness. Much of this depends upon the bicarbonates of lime and magnesia in solution and on the presence of free CO_2.

672. Now, in boiling water for half an hour the heat dissipates the CO_2 and transforms the bicarbonates into simple carbonates, which being insoluble are precipitated. This leaves certain soluble lime and magnesia compounds (usually sulphates) which cannot be extracted. The temporary hardness has been removed and the permanent hardness remains.

673. Or, in a small way, add carbonate of soda (washing-soda). The reaction leads to bicarbonate of soda and carbonate of lime. The soda bicarbonate is soluble, but the insoluble lime carbonate is precipitated. This is the domestic practice in the laundry.

674. Or, the third and best method, known as Clark's process, which depends on the addition of lime. This is applied on a large scale, the quantity of lime being determined by the soap test. The lime subtracts a certain amount of CO_2 from the soluble bicarbonate of lime, converting it into an insoluble carbonate, which, with the carbonate originally present, falls to the bottom.

675. When there are 20–30 parts bicarbonate of lime per 100,000, about 9 oz. quicklime is used to every 400 gals. of water, or 1 gal. clear lime-water to every 10 gals. of water   Used on a large scale,

as in certain British cities whose water is peculiarly adapted to it, besides improving the quality of the water for the table, a great economic saving is made in the consumption of soap.

SUSPENDED MATTERS AND THEIR REMOVAL.

Sedimentation.

676. Water may contain in suspension as well as in solution both organic and mineral matter, and it is against this suspended matter, which is offensive to the eye, that the most of the processes of clarification and filtration are directed.

677. Muddy water usually contains insoluble particles of slightly greater specific gravity than the water itself, and when allowed to rest sedimentation will free it from most of the foreign matters, and, speaking generally, the remainder can usually be removed by straining. Settling-basins on a large scale are therefore important adjuncts to reservoirs.

678. But, excepting diarrhœa from mechanical irritation, mud, although unsightly, rarely causes disease. This diarrhœa, however, sometimes is grave and persistent. Settling, by rest, on a small scale is often efficacious for domestic use, so that water as muddy as the Missouri will become perfectly clear if allowed to remain undisturbed for twenty-four hours in a convenient vessel. The suspended alluvium falls to the bottom and the supernatant liquid can be poured off.

679. Suspended matters are also removed by precipitation and filtration.

Precipitation.

680. Precipitation is sedimentation either by rest (as just described), or through clarification, which, by inducing harmless chemical changes, leads to it.

681. The most convenient agent for precipitation, especially if the water is slightly hard, is alum. Add about 6 grains of crystallized alum to the gallon or move about in the water a lump of alum held in the hand. Some years ago, one wing of a British regiment passing up the Indus drank the water without preparation and suffered severely from a diarrhœa of irritation. The other wing used alum and had no diarrhœa. The first then adopted it and the diarrhœa ceased.

682. Should the water be very soft, first introduce a little calcium chloride and sodium carbonate. The rationale is the formation of calcium sulphate from calcium carbonate, which, together with the bulky aluminum hydrate, entangles the suspended particles and sinks with them.

683. Other methods are: The use of perchloride of iron, 1 oz. to 250 gals., following it by $2\frac{3}{4}$ oz. carbonate of soda to neutralize the acidity and remove the excess of iron.

684. Cactus-leaves cut up have a clarifying effect.

Other Methods of Purification.

685. Citric acid, 1 oz. to 16 gals., improves water by its action on contained minute vegetable growths (algæ). Tannin in small quantities does the same; but when tannin is used the water should stand

some hours. Growing vegetation, although the water may be colored green thereby, is usually of advantage; but dead vegetation may do harm.

686. A solution of permanganate of potassium (Condy's fluid), a teaspoonful at a time added to 3 or 4 gallons of water until a slight permanent pink color is obtained, followed by 6 grains crystallized alum to the gallon, removes the disagreeable odor of impure water in casks.

687. The action of the permanganate is that of an oxidizer. After having lost much of its reputation, it has again come into favor in India as a preventive of cholera. Enough (an ounce or more) should be dissolved in a well to insure a reddish tinge for twenty-four hours. In excess it kills contained animal life and thus spoils the water. (Harrington, after Hankin, *Ind. Med. Gaz.*, July, 1896.)

688. Schumburg (*Deut. med. Woch.*, 4th Mar., 1897), according to Harrington, claims that all pathogenic bacteria in water are killed in five minutes by 1 cc. of a 20 per cent. solution of bromine and potassic bromide, each, to 5 litres ordinary river-water. In very hard or grossly polluted water more of the solution should be added gradually until a yellow tinge, that will persist half a minute, occurs. Under any circumstances, a volume of 9 per cent. ammonia solution equal to that of the bromine solution must be added.

689. The bromine method, which appears to be trustworthy, is particularly adapted to the military service either for small parties or for large commands. A kilogram (2.2 lbs.) of bromine will sterilize 16,000 litres (3500 gals.) of common water.

690. Where circumstances permit, as on steamships, at posts, and in some camps, distillation will sterilize the drinking-water. But if the source of supply is very impure, certain impurities may be carried over with the steam, and these may induce diarrhœas.

691. Thorough boiling, which is nearly always practicable, even in active campaign, efficiently destroys the bacterial causes of disease, and should be employed for all drinking-water when there is any doubt of its purity.

Filtration.

692. Filtration is directed against suspended matters, dissolved organic matter, and bacterial organisms.

693. Filters have three modes of action:

(1) By mechanically arresting suspended matter too large to pass through their pores; that is, by straining. (2) By the attraction of masses, as when water passing very slowly through a filter makes deposits in the interstices. (3) By the removal of substances actually dissolved in the water.

694. On a large scale a sand-filter consists of fine sand superimposed upon coarse sand, which rests upon fine gravel, and that in turn on coarse gravel. When properly constructed and managed, this is very efficient in almost completely removing the bacterial and other organic causes of disease. But these filters are so costly in their construction and care as to make them available only for large communities.

695. Such a filter restrains gross impurities mechanically, but its most valuable function is the nitrification of organic matter and the destruction of microbes. This is effected in a gelatinous layer that forms in the upper part of the filter, the living matter of which is the efficient agent. As the free surfaces of the particles of sand are out of all apparent proportion to the cubical bulk of the mass, there is a very large area upon which the so-called "bacterial jelly" is formed. Such a filter becomes clogged or "dead" at irregular intervals, when it requires renovation by scraping and washing the removed sand.

696. When cistern-water must be filtered for a house supply, it should pass over a chamber that would retain the coarse sediment and then be conducted under a layer of coarse gravel that supports one of sand, through which it percolates upward. The sand must be renewed every three or four months.

697. A simpler tank filter is where the filtering material is raised a few inches from the bottom, leaving a settling-basin from which the water passes upward.

698. It is a fundamental principle that every filter, whether fixed or movable, should be accessible in all its parts, for none is automatic in its renovating power.

699. Portable filters are usually designed to restrain the impurities mechanically.

700. Animal charcoal (bone-black), formerly supposed very efficient, is really objectionable in that it yields phosphates and N, which favor the growth of

bacteria in water. It oxidizes putrefactive organic matter, but permits active organic matter to pass through unchanged. In other words, it does not sterilize the water but is liable to make it more hurtful. Thus after a month's use the filtrate contained five times as many germs as the unfiltered water.

701. Vegetable charcoal, or coke, makes an efficient filter against micro-organisms (P. Frankland), but should be frequently renewed.

702. Spongy iron arrests suspended matter and oxidizes organic matter. It appears to deteriorate very slowly, and therefore to require renewal. Frankland says after one month's action it detains 99.8 per cent. of micro-organisms. Notter and Firth say it permits the free passage of bacteria.

703. Sponge, sometimes used in individual filters, acts only mechanically, and is objectionable as being itself organic, and very soon becomes foul. Cotton and wool, whether woven or in their natural state, are bad for the same reason.

704. Asbestos, if arranged so that it may be treated with fire and replaced, is much better material for an individual filter.

705. The best filter hitherto devised for domestic use is unglazed porcelain, through which the water passes under moderate pressure. This acts mechanically but efficiently, entirely sterilizing the water. The most efficient form is the Chamberland-Pasteur. As the bacteria will ultimately grow through the kaolin, the "candle" (bougie) must be removed weekly, and be carefully brushed and boiled, or be well heated in a flame. It is absolutely efficient under those conditions.

706. The Berkefeld filter is of the same general type as the Chamberland, with tubes assembled in a battery. Turbid water should first be clarified, as it soon coats the outside of the cylinders and reduces the yield. Under 40 pounds pressure 15 cylinders will yield 7½ gals., and 3 cylinders 1½ gals., a minute. Constant attention is needed both to boil and to scour the tubes, and as these are fragile, the filter's utility depends very much upon the care with which it is operated. Under normal conditions it is excellent; with careless men it soon deteriorates.

707. The official sterilizer supplied the army is the Forbes-Waterhouse, whose efficiency depends on the action of heat and its economy of operation upon its conservation of that force. It is believed that it destroys all living organisms.

708. A good field filter is a cask charred on the inside (that may occasionally be brushed) and pierced with very small holes through the bottom. This is sunk in the water, which will rise through the holes. Better is one barrel within another, the outer pierced through the bottom and the inner near the top, the intervening space being filled with sand, gravel, or similar material, and the whole sunk sufficiently in the stream.

Water as a Disease-bearer.

709. Several grave diseases are intimately associated with water as a cause-bearer, if not as a cause. These are cholera, typhoid fever, and a variety of dysentery, which are spread by discharges from in-

fected persons that, as a rule, gain access to the new victims with food and drink. Their most common mode of propagation is through the contaminated drinking-water.

710. It has not been demonstrated that typhoid fever may originate from sewage not specifically poisoned; but it is certain that both it and cholera are caused by their specific excreta. And as both typhoid fever and cholera begin with a painless diarrhœa whose import the invalid does not understand, it is quite possible for such discharges to drain into any but the best-kept water-supply, so that epidemics of great magnitude sometimes begin in this way.

711. A well-authenticated example, among many others, is that where, in 1885, the washing of the discharges of a single case from the bank of a stream, into the stream itself that supplied water to a town of 8000 inhabitants, was followed by an epidemic of 1104 cases of typhoid fever, resulting in 114 deaths and great loss of time and labor.

712. Two factories that employed many hands stood side by side, but the men drank from two distinct wells. One of these wells was pure and the other was believed to be infected. Of those who drank from the infected well, 600 died of cholera, but of the others, none.

713. A severe and fatal variety of dysentery has repeatedly been traced to impure water; water not recognized as charged with dysenteric products, but contaminated with fæcal impurities. And widespread diarrhœas have ceased when the general water-supply has been changed to one that is purer.

On the other hand, water known to be specifically contaminated spreads dysentery with facility.

714. Water that is contaminated with animal waste is not necessarily disagreeable; it is apt to be more sparkling and may be very pleasant. And although no one would willingly drink sewage, nevertheless sewage-tainted wells may not induce disease. But the sewage in them is at any time liable to have a specific taint imparted without changing their physical characteristics.

715. Such water is sometimes more clear and palatable than that in good wells, and it often is difficult to persuade those accustomed to use it of the truth, or to make them understand how leakage may enter over long and unsuspected routes. The worst supplies in fact—not in appearance—are the unsuspected, for had they been suspected their use would not have been persisted in.

716. As examples of contamination at a distance: A well nearly free from iron suddenly began to yield chalybeate water, which deposited an ochreous sediment. It proved that a quantity of spoiled beer having been emptied into the ground 115 feet from the well, its organic matter acted as a reducing agent on ferric oxide in the soil, which dissolving as a protocarbonate entered the water that supplied the well. This might as well have been infected sewage. Gas from a main 1000 feet away has been recognized in well-water. The typhoid poison has been conveyed several miles by an underground flow, as at Lausen in 1872.

717. The peculiar liability of limestone regions to fissures and subterranean caverns, through which

water freely communicates over long distances, makes them eminently subject to the spread of cholera.

718. Specific disease-causes may not be extracted by filtration, nor respond to chemical tests, nor be antagonized by chemical agents, at least so that the water remains potable. But there are chemical indications by which sewage may be suspected, such as the presence of chlorides, of nitrates, of nitrites.

719. Should a suspected well materially differ chemically from neighboring wells, it is probably infected. In that case the chemical condition is a sign, not a cause. Of course a chain of wells may be similarly affected, in which case special investigation must be made.

720. The simplest way to determine whether a communicating channel exists, is to introduce into the cesspool or other suspected locality a quantity of salt or brine and later to observe what change, if any, there is in the chlorides in the well. If they have increased, the inference that the contents of the privy may enter the well is obvious. Lithia, which is not found in ordinary soils, is a more delicate test.

721. When chlorides in excess, the nitrates, and the nitrites are reported they are to be looked upon as derived from sewage or similar filth, unless there are plain indications of their origin from perfectly innocent sources. By themselves, like CO_2 in the air, unless in enormous quantities, they are harmless; but they are an index of possible mischief, and point to typhoid fever, cholera, or sometimes dysentery, in the water-supply, if consumers of it have such a disease.

722. The ordinary domestic rural well may be poisoned by infection making its way through the ground, especially along rifts; but it is more apt to be thus charged, as Sedgwick claims, from the top. Loosely-covered wells may be polluted in numerous ways, the opportunities multiplying with the density of the population and the age of the settlement. But until specifically infected, it will cause no specific disease. The military application here is to remote posts, and to the marches and camps of real and mimic war.

723. It is manifestly unwise to assume that infected dejecta discharged upon the ground or buried in it will be neutralized before reaching a neighboring well, especially as it is impossible to determine that there is no rift in the soil allowing direct communication. But the best authorities regard the chance of indirect infection as very small.

724. Nevertheless, Vaughan has discovered organic matter in the soil on nearly level ground 50 feet from a privy-vault, by comparison with other soil of the same kind where there were no known sources of contamination; and such matter might be infected.

725. The typhoid cause may persist in unfiltered water for thirty days, but usually perishes much sooner. The cholera cause has a relatively short life in water, except as reinforced from without. In the presence of saprophytes, pathogenic bacteria generally disappear quickly in contaminated water. Where a sand-filter is used these specific organisms become entangled in the "bacterial jelly."

726. Doubtless in most cases of water infection the cause is a continuing one, following the addition of

new material, which should be sought out and prevented. It is, however, much better to avoid the original pollution of water-supply than to depend upon removing the poison once introduced.

727. Independently of the specific disease-poisons intimately associated with water-carriage, there are non-specific impurities, generally held in suspension but sometimes in solution. Organic remains in water are always impurities, never being present naturally, as in some sense the minerals that are in solution might be regarded. These may come from animal waste or even from animal decomposition, as in the soakage of graveyards, and from vegetable decay.

728. But in view of the inconceivable amount of organic disintegration going on through all time, why is not all water a mere vehicle to carry this waste? Because the free oxygen in the soil and in the water allows unrestrained oxidation, and because certain minute organisms associated generally with mineral matter and known as the bacteria of nitrification decompose the waste, freeing ammonia. Then from this ammonia, nitric acid and subsequently the nitrites and nitrates are formed.

729. The nitrites and nitrates therefore are indications that animal waste has been present in the water. When waste has reached that stage its power for evil has gone, but more waste may follow too rapidly for the soil to neutralize; or it may be there already in excess.

730. Concentrated waste in the shape of sewage must ultimately overcome the regenerating influences of a limited area, and these indications of pre-exist-

ing danger should lead to the suspicion of present danger.

731. The preceding chiefly concerns wells toward which broken sewers or imperfect vaults may ooze, or down whose mouths surface slops may drip.

The Detection of Organic Waste in Water.

732. The presence, not the amount, of organic matter may be roughly determined thus:

Half fill a quart bottle with water at 70°–80° F.; shake it vigorously, and if a bad odor is detected it is doubtful or bad. But all bad waters do not have an odor. Therefore evaporate 3 or 4 ounces to perfect dryness in a porcelain or platinum capsule, and then ignite the dish. If there is no blackening or only an easily-dissipated darkening of the residue, the water is probably good. If the crust blackens, there is probably carbon from an excess of vegetation. If nitrous fumes are evolved and the carbon sparkles with energy, animal matter may be suspected.

733. The permanganate salts are rich in oxygen that is easily given up. Permanganate of potash added by degrees until the oxygen is absorbed colors water a rich pink or red. From the amount required to tinge the water an estimate may be made of the quantity, but not of the kind, of organic matter. It responds equally to beef soup and street filth.

The Ultimate Disappearance of Sewage.

734. What becomes of the vast quantity of sewage poured into running streams—often those that sooner or later furnish drinking-water for communities,

although no community should risk taking its drinking-water from such a stream?

735. It is commonly said that streams purify themselves. Dilution has much to do with the apparent disappearance of sewage; the volume of water is very great, and the sewage becomes immensely attenuated. But even specific organic particles do disappear in some way, and the accumulation of deadly poison, that *a priori* would seem necessary, does not occur.

736. As a rule immediately, and always finally, subsoil water tends toward the river-courses. It either swells the river by its direct volume, which is the reason why a stream increases as it descends, independently of tributaries, or it forms a subaqueous river. In most cases both conditions exist.

737. This constant addition of practically uncontaminated ground-water steadily dilutes any given amount of sewage. All water holds in solution some oxygen, which does its part in oxidation. Where there are rapids probably more oxygen is entangled, but, contrary to the older opinion, it has been found that swiftly-running water does not purify itself as quickly as that which is still. The immersed solid matter is acted on by the bacteria of decomposition; sedimentation takes place literally, or practically by the suspended silt enveloping the particles of sewage. Light and vegetation are active agents. But with it all, Mason believes that the percentage of pollution to disappear per mile of flow continually decreases as the stream advances.

738. The discharge of sewage into streams whose banks are inhabited should be forbidden by law, as

it now is in England and in some parts of this country.

Water-supply for Troops.

739. On halting for even a temporary camp the water-supply must be immediately guarded, and with special precaution if it is small. Great care should be taken that the margin of a stream is not trampled into mud and the water made turbid. To this end it is profitable immediately to lay down an approach, as of rails, boards, or logs. Wells should be protected against both pollution and waste.

740. By moderately digging out a small spring and sinking a casing or barrel, the visible supply will be increased and waste avoided. If the stream is shallow, promptly make a small reservoir by a temporary dam for drinking, one below for the horses, and one still lower for washing. Horses will drink better and more rapidly where the water is 5 or 6 inches deep, which can easily be arranged. Where it is limited, an officer should be in immediate charge of the whole water-supply.

741. At a permanent camp where the command is large in proportion to the water-supply, make one or more reservoirs to retain the water that flows by night and draw from them the cooking- and drinking-water. Extend lower down a single or double row of sunken half-barrels for horses, all connected by little gutters to avoid waste, and conduct the surplus into a still lower reservoir.

742. An essay for the use of volunteers, published in 1861, advised placing latrines over running water when possible. Fortunately this was corrected in

the next edition, and it is only cited to show that the importance of guarding water is sometimes strangely overlooked (*Ref. Hd. Bk. Med. Sci.*, 1st ed., III, p. 756). Munson reports that precisely the same error was committed by raw troops in the late Spanish war. (See par. 509.)

743. "Nothing is better established than that no refuse, and especially no fæcal matter, should be discharged so as to follow a stream either directly or indirectly, unless it be one of the great rivers, and then only when it is certain that the water is to be used by no one within a reasonable distance. It is suicidal to pollute small streams that may possibly supply our own forces, then or later, and it is criminal to spread disease in that way among a civil population, or . . . to an enemy." (*Ref. Hd. Bk.*, *loc. cit.*)

744. On the march a man requires for cooking and drinking 6 pints a day, increased in hot climates to 8 pints, and an equal amount for washing the person. In stationary camps 5 gals. for all purposes. In barracks, for all purposes except water-closets and bath-rooms, 10 gals. per head. With water-closets and baths, 25 gals. Hospitals require several times as much per man, depending on the character of the cases.

745. A horse drinks about 1½ gals., requiring three minutes. Each gulp represents about 3 ounces. Horses, if allowed all they will drink, require 6–10 gals. per day, and about 3 gals. per head for police purposes. All the foregoing figures are the lowest.

Snow and Ice.

746. Snow is more impure than rain from the same region. It takes up foreign substances freely from the air through which it passes and absorbs them from the soil on which it lies. Snow-water, especially in densely inhabited regions, equally with other doubtful water, should be boiled before consumption.

747. Water is partly purified by freezing, but so imperfectly as to require the sources of ice-supply for domestic use to be as carefully selected and guarded as those of water.

748. Clear ice from polluted sources may contain a very small proportion of injurious matter; but snow-ice and that obtained by flooding is apt to be unsafe. As bacteria are attracted by air-bubbles, "bubbly ice" is especially dangerous.

749. Artificial ice, unless from distilled water, may be more impure than natural ice from the same water.

VIII.

PREVENTABLE DISEASES.

Malaria.

750. Malaria, literally bad air, has gradually come to mean a disease or a class of diseases. It is distinctly recognized that a parasitic micro-organism found in the blood, known as the *plasmodium malariæ*, is so closely associated with it that this must be regarded as the cause.

751. These *plasmodia* have not yet been isolated outside of living bodies, and their absolute origin is not known. But it has been clearly demonstrated that for them the variety of mosquito known as *anopheles*, whether single or multiple, but probably multiple, acts an intermediate host, and that the parasite completes its development in the red corpuscles of the human blood.

752. The disease is spread by the mosquito sucking from the blood of a malarial patient the parasite which, after several stages within the insect, reaches its salivary glands, whence it enters the new subject that may be bitten.

753. Hence if one is not bitten by an infected mosquito he will not contract the disease. Therefore the immediate precaution is to preserve the person by the careful use of netting, or to repel the

174

insect for the time by the application to exposed parts of the person of pungent aromatic oils, as pennyroyal or eucalyptus.

754. Within a barrack or other dwelling, mosquitoes resting on the ceiling, and sometimes those on the walls, may be destroyed by cautiously holding under them a small vessel (as the top of a tin can on the end of a light pole) containing a little household ammonia, mineral oil, or spirits of turpentine. Any of these vapors stupefies the insect and it falls into the cup.

755. The mosquito may be exterminated by drying up the pools, often very small, mere footprints in the ground, or emptying cans containing a little water, in which they breed, and by killing the larvæ by a film of mineral oil over such water as cannot be removed. The mosquitoes that hibernate are usually impregnated female *anopheles*, and Giles, quoted by Abbott, "makes the valuable suggestion that during the hibernating season all buildings likely to harbor the impregnated *anopheles* [particularly the eaves of barns, houses, and outbuildings, as well as their interiors] should be thoroughly renovated, lime-washed, and fumigated with sulphur," to which may be added, or with formaldehyde or the fumes of burning pyrethrum (insect-powder), or even tobacco or the smoke of green wood.

756. According to the present state of our knowledge, malarial disease would be abolished if all infected mosquitoes were exterminated and all malarial patients were made well by the destruction, through the systematic use of quinine, of the parasites within the body, so as to cut off the supply of infecting material.

757. By no means all *anopheles* are infected, for they are found over large areas quite untainted; but they may become infected when they feed on malarial patients. And such patients, perhaps not very susceptible to its immediate effects, yield a constant supply of the poison. For instance, in nearly all Filipino scouts, even when apparently well, the parasite is present, and from them the insect readily transfers it to the associated white soldiers.

758. In like manner infected immigrants have introduced the disease for the first time into an isolated and hitherto immune country, whence practically the whole population was attacked, as in the Island of Mauritius about 1865.

759. Although not yet isolated outside of human or insect life, the virulence of the poison notoriously varies in different regions. It is peculiarly deadly in some places, and such localities should be carefully avoided, either as camping-places or merely to be marched through.

760. Notwithstanding all direct experiment to convey the disease by drinking water taken from malarious marshes has failed, there is a widely established belief that such water may induce the disease. In deference thereto the use of boiled water, preferably as tea or coffee, is commended.

761. There is little doubt that a well-nourished and properly clad person resists malarial disease, even when the cause enters the blood, better than the weak.

762. Whether it is exclusively an attribute of insect life or not, it remains true that whatever the

nature of the malarial poison, it appears to be borne for limited distances by the wind, to lie comparatively near the ground, to be stopped by mechanical barriers, to be avoided by residence in an upper story, and to take effect most distinctly when the exposed person is poorly nourished, ill-clad, and with an empty stomach, and the danger of infection is greater at night. All these conditions are satisfied by the mosquito theory.

Typhoid Fever and Cholera.

763. Typhoid fever is strictly an eruptive disease, and like other eruptive diseases is unlikely to attack the same person twice. As it is very likely to prevail among newly-raised troops, the utmost caution is required to avoid its propagation, which chiefly occurs through the discharges from the bowels and the kidneys. In camp all fæcal discharges should be thoroughly disposed of, because it is impossible at the outset to distinguish a typhoid-fever case from a simple diarrhœa.

764. In poorly conserved camps it is very possible for polluted dust to convey the disease by being swallowed with food or otherwise. And it has been demonstrated that flies will convey upon their feet the infecting matter from the dejecta to food. (See par. 515.)

765. This general conclusion of the Washington Medical Committee is unimpeachable: Typhoid fever increases in proportion to the saturation of the soil with decomposing organic matter, especially human excreta, and to the drinking of infected well-water.

766. Our exact knowledge as to the life of the typhoid germ in the soil when undisturbed is not satisfactory. It is believed that it is not destroyed by the oxidizing and nitrifying bacteria, and authorities assign it a vitality ranging from two days to six months. This variation probably depends on the character of the soil.

767. Cholera has nothing in common with typhoid fever except its tendency to spread through the discharges, especially from the bowels. It may occur several times in the same person. But mild or "walking" cases of typhoid fever and those of choleraic diarrhœa, for both diseases at the beginning have their only indication of sickness in a painless diarrhœa, are very liable to infect communities.

768. The cholera cause probably escapes change in the soil for a considerable period when only influenced by natural causes, wherein it is like the typhoid cause, but it has a relatively short life in water except as reinforced from without. The utmost caution is necessary in disinfecting the discharges of both cholera and typhoid fever before disposing of them, and in preserving the water-supply from contamination.

769. For the same reason old camp-grounds, and especially those once infected, are always condemned. But neither cholera nor typhoid fever is contagious by mere presence, as smallpox is.

770. It is probable that the cholera poison does not flourish in acid fluids either within or without the body, and both of these diseases spread more easily where alkaline fermentation occurs. Hence

to acidulate the excreta is one of the best preventives against these diseases spreading.

771. Carbolic acid in excess, sulphate of iron (copperas), or, best of all, mercuric bichloride (corrosive sublimate) are to be used for every discharge, including the urine in typhoid fever and the vomit in cholera, which must be thoroughly disinfected before committal to the sewers. But mercuric bichloride corrodes metals, and it should not be passed through lead or iron pipes.

772. Should there be no sewers, similar disinfection must be practised and the whole be buried beyond any possible contamination of air or water. Everything contaminated by excreta of any kind in these diseases is to be similarly and completely disinfected or destroyed.

773. There is no known chemical method of antagonizing the typhoid poison in water, so as to leave it fit to drink. But Munson quotes Christmas as saying that 0.6–0.8 gm. citric or tartaric acid to the litre surely sterilizes water against the cholera cause. This is perfectly harmless and is not disagreeable.

774. Should there be danger of an outbreak of cholera, in the absence of direct medical advice it would be well in addition to boiling the water to put the command on an acidulated drink, as "lemonade" of aromatic sulphuric acid. This is believed to have prevented the disease in special communities.

775. Protective "vaccination," so called, more strictly inoculation by proper toxins, has been employed on a large scale and with fair success against typhoid fever, cholera, and plague.

Yellow Fever.

776. Yellow fever is a disease of navigable regions in hot and moist climates that, as a rule, does not twice attack the same person. Walter Reed has demonstrated both positively and negatively that it is propagated, and propagated only, by the mosquito. The female of the *Stegomyia fasciata* is the intermediate host for the specific agent of this disease, as the *anopheles* is for the malarial cause. Like the latter, it has not yet been demonstrated out of living bodies. The *Stegomyia* is essentially a domestic mosquito, not flying afield like the *anopheles* and *culex*.

777. The prevention of yellow fever consists in destroying the mosquitoes that have been or may become infected. Gorgas has proved the possibility of doing this, even in so vast and fertile a hotbed as Havana. No mosquito should be allowed to reach a yellow-fever patient, nor, having become infected, to escape from the apartment.

778. This disease may be avoided, speaking generally, by removing the troops to a locality, such as can usually be found not remote from the seat of outbreak, where it will not spread. Presumably this immunity is due to the absence of the special mosquito.

779. The sick person and the infected mosquito, not the effects nor the quarters of the sick, alone spread the disease. It develops in man within five days after infection. If, therefore, non-immunes who have been exposed are detained five days and do not sicken, they may safely be admitted.

780. The infection develops within the mosquito in twelve days, after which time the insect is capable of conveying the disease by its bite Therefore the most rigorous exclusion must be maintained against possibly infected insects through fumigation directed against all manner of containers, from ships and railroad-cars to hand-bags and open cans. Disinfection by germicides is superfluous, but to destroy the insect is imperative.

781. With the opening of an Isthmian canal, the utmost caution must be used against receiving infected insects on shipboard within our own tropics and conveying them to Asia, where the disease has never occurred. The *Stegomyia*, not yet infected, abounds in the Philippines.

Plague.

782. Plague, practically confined under our flag to the Oriental races, is nevertheless always a possible menace to our troops in the Philippines. Its cause is a bacillus introduced through a break in the skin. This flourishes best in filthy soil, although of course filth does not originate it, and it is carried over wide areas by vermin, especially by mice and rats.

783. Cleanliness of person and of surroundings is an element of protection. Rats, its great distributors, should be exterminated as far as possible. And a preventive toxin may be used.

Consumption and Diphtheria.

784. Consumption depends upon a bacillus disseminated not by the breath but by the sputa which are charged with it. When the sputa are sufficiently

dried to be blown about they may be inhaled, and the contained bacilli, if not destroyed in the blood, set up the disease. In proportion as a barrack or other apartment is crowded, is there the risk of this disease spreading from any accidentally introduced case; and the risk diminishes exactly as the air-space enlarges. Nearly all armies that were formerly ravaged by consumption are now practically exempt, owing to their greater air allowance in barracks.

785. In the army every recognized consumptive is immediately transferred to a special post, where the best sanitary arrangements for combating the disease prevail. As soon as the sputum in any protracted "cold" becomes yellow, it should be examined microscopically for the bacillus, and when that is found the soldier should be transferred. All infected sputa should be passed into a combustible spit-cup and be kept moist, and the cup and the handkerchiefs be burned, the man should be comparatively isolated, and his special apartment must be disinfected.

786. It must be carefully remembered that consumption progresses so rapidly at the ocean-level in the Philippines that immediate removal is imperative—either to the interior mountain land or, better, to the United States.

787. Diphtheria is an eminently infectious disease also depending upon a bacillus which enters the air-passages, not from the patient's breath but with minute particles of false membrane dislodged by coughing or sneezing. It clings persistently to places where once established; its spread is greatly fostered by foul air and imperfect ventilation; and disinfec-

tion should be active and complete. A preventive antitoxin, administered subcutaneously to healthy persons directly exposed to the disease, will protect against diphtheria for a limited period.

Contagious Diseases and Disinfectants.

788. Measles and mumps are contagious diseases that almost every person has at some period of life. There is no known method of preventing them except by avoiding their presence, which is generally impossible. As these are serious in camp, special hospital provision must be made among newly-raised troops. (See par. 90.)

789. Scarlet fever and smallpox are not inevitable diseases, but are contagious and when they occur are very serious. Smallpox is always to be restrained among the well by preventive vaccination.

790. The direct contagion of scarlet fever is not strong, but its persistence is extreme, even after years of burial, and the disease itself is very grave, especially in northern latitudes. Everything connected with such a case—clothing, toys, and especially books—should be burned. Infected rooms and houses are to be thoroughly scraped, lime-washed, painted, and scrubbed with corrosive sublimate 1:1000, as well as be absolutely ventilated. Small wooden houses about a post it is safer to destroy by fire.

791. "A disinfectant is an agent capable of destroying the infective power of infectious material." Substances that merely neutralize bad odors are not disinfectants; they are deodorants.

792. The best disinfectants are "dry and moist heat; sulphur dioxide; the hypochlorites of lime and

of soda (chloride of lime and Labarraque's solution); mercuric chloride; cupric sulphate; carbolic acid" (Sternberg); and sunlight.

793. Formaldehyde, generated by the action of heat (from a special lamp) on wood alcohol, in the presence of moisture, is an efficient germicide for exposed micro-organisms. It will not penetrate fabrics deeply. It kills mosquitoes only when brought into direct contact with sufficient concentration.

794. "It is impracticable to disinfect an occupied apartment," but it should be carefully closed and 3 pounds of sulphur be burned in it for every 1000 cubic feet. It must afterward be washed down by hand with a solution of 1 to 1000 of corrosive sublimate, 2 to 100 of carbolic acid, or 1 to 100 of chloride of lime or sulphate of iron. (Am. Pub. Health Assoc.)

795. For privy-vaults use 1 pound corrosive sublimate dissolved in much water, to 500 pounds estimated contents of vault.

In Conclusion.

796. Finally, the efficient care of troops is a work full of prosaic detail, but the minutiæ expand naturally so that the care of an armed man and that of an army are problems of similar factors, only varying in their power, in the science of military hygiene.

797. Besides their physical care, the cultivation of contentment and judicious appeals to personal and professional pride are important in forming the best soldiers.

IX.

THE CARE OF TROOPS IN THE FIELD.

The very first fact in the efficiency of an army is its health. The success of a campaign depends upon hostile contact, actual as in battle or potential as in manœuvres; but in either form those operations require vigorous men for their execution. As every student of military affairs knows, the deaths in the field from disease far exceed those from the casualties of action, and the discharges for disability for illness greatly outnumber those for wounds. It is also true that the newer the troops the more sickly are they, so that sometimes the ranks are much reduced before the enemy is found. That is, it is the camp and not the battle that at first and most seriously disables men. The prevention of very much of this disease lies in the hands of officers of the line. Medical officers can point out the methods of prevention, but their execution rests with the officers in actual command. By an intelligent application of their authority these can reduce the preventable disease to the minimum, and nearly all camp disease is preventable.

A large improvised army of seasoned troops is a contradiction of terms. Therefore when a newly-raised army is to take the field, its material should be selected as carefully as possible. Youthful recruits have little military value. Men for active service

185

should not be less than twenty-two years of age, or they would be too immature physiologically. Immature men in the ranks require special care, because their endurance and adaptability are inferior as a class. Such soldiers succumb under the exertion and hardships that at any time may, and sometimes must, be required of them.

All collections of young men are liable to epidemics of such contagious diseases as measles, mumps, German measles, scarlet fever, as they may not have suffered from in childhood; on which account rural recruits in particular furnish a large immediate sick-list. Regiments raised directly in the country must expect to pass through a period of inefficiency from measles alone. That disease always ravages such commands. It is a very serious matter for adults in camp, and the colder the climate the more grave are its consequences. There is practically no way except by isolation to prevent these contagious diseases. The most that regimental officers can do is to provide abundant air-space and protection against the weather for those within range.

Rural recruits do not bear as well as those from the towns the irregular hours and the night work of military life, nor do they learn as quickly. But after they have become habituated to discipline and its requirements they are more efficient.

All recruits are apt to suffer from troubles of digestion and assimilation. The plainer food and, particularly, the cooking with which in the beginning they are supplied disturb the health of many, and one of the first duties of a company commander is to secure a really competent field cook for his men. Intelligent assistants should then be detailed in succession, so as to spread a knowledge of the preparation of food as rapidly as possible. When every man can acceptably cook his own ration under the conditions of the bivouac, that command has reached a high state of efficiency. It is in this respect that volunteers, and especially the organized militia, are often woefully at fault. When called into service they do not know how to prepare their food. Training of this kind, instead of dependence upon hired caterers in their summer camps, would add immeasurably to their efficiency when first mustered in. The National Guard should understand that military cooking is more important than markmanship in the early days of a campaign. It is useless to place in front of the enemy, or indeed to hold in reserve, men however well equipped who cannot keep the field in vigor from inability to subsist on the food supplied. On account of the common difficulty with field food at the beginning, an extra supply of good bread should always be provided. It is invariably acceptable to recruits, it is a good diet, and none of it goes to waste.

The most important single article of uniform is the shoe, and it is a company officer's duty to see that his men are properly equipped in that way as soon as they are mustered in. The soldier's marching capacity depends upon the character of his footgear, and it is also in this respect that the organized militia when mustered in with State equipment are apt to be defective, because so many of those men wear their civilian's shoe under military conditions. One of the most painful trials for all troops beginning a campaign, whether otherwise trained or not, is foot-soreness. The almost invariable attempt of raw troops to make an excessive march in every-day shoes leads to a great deal of agony that might be avoided. The military shoe as issued is not ideal, but it is much better than what the soldier will buy and wear if not prevented. No man should be excused from wearing the regulation shoe, unless under very exceptional circumstances certified by a medical officer of experience. To be serviceable, a marching-shoe should be large enough in all directions, but not too large. When the foot moves within the shoe it is quite apt to develop chafes. The shoes should be made supple with oil, and for better endurance have hobnails in the sole. The company officer should convince himself by direct and repeated personal inspection that his men's feet are properly cared for as to nails, and in the absence of corns and bunions. Men should be instructed to cut the nails square across, not rounded, a *little* but not too far behind the end of the toe. Especially when there is a tendency to grow in, the corner of the nail must not be rounded.

Before a march the foot should be well greased with tallow or neat's-foot oil (but these are not easily had in the field), or the inside of the stocking should be covered with a stiff lather, carefully rubbed in, of common yellow soap (which always should be at hand). Should the stockings excite pain on a prolonged march, the pressure is sometimes relieved by changing them to the other feet or by turning them inside out. Plain rags wrapped around the feet are an efficient substitute for stockings, that sometimes are very comfortable and always are much cleaner. A blister on the foot should be opened by only a prick at the lowest point. Or, better if practicable, pass a threaded needle through it and tie the ends of the thread together. This will drain the fluid without disturbing the delicate skin. The next day the ends of the thread may be cut off, but the inner part should not be removed. To soak the feet in water, especially cold water, although grateful at the time, is of doubtful advantage. It is better to wipe them carefully with a damp towel or to bathe them gently with tepid water and rub in an animal oil. The latter is hardly practicable on a march. Chafed and inflamed surfaces should be well greased or be covered with a clay poultice (Sundberg). The salicylic and talcum foot-powder or ointment within the stocking is particularly efficacious. Spare stockings should be put on at the end of the march, and those worn during the day be dried and beaten, or if possible be washed, for the morrow.

Individual cleanliness is a material factor of health and efficiency, and the stated inspections by company officers should embrace the condition of the person and of the underclothing. At least once a week at an inspection, combined with the daily inspection of quarters or not, the actual condition should be observed under commands similar to these: "Remove both shoes and one stocking! Open coats and shirts! Non-commi sioned officers excepted." Uncleanliness thus observed should be followed up. An inspection confined to the outer dress and satisfied with clean spare underclothing in the blanket-roll, regardless of what may be on the

person, is unworthy the name and encourages con-
cealment. This is the more important with new
troops, because with some of them exact care of the
person is an unfamiliar task and to all the meagre
accommodations of the field interpose obstacles.
Recruits require nearly as much supervisory care as
children, and it should be given unremittingly and
intelligently until they become adapted to their
new life. On that account, that they may see as
well as hear what to do, it is very desirable to assign
regular recruits to organized companies as promptly
as they are sufficiently drilled not to destroy the formation. And it is equally important to introduce
a few good old soldiers, if they can be found, into
volunteer organizations. The exception is never
to use a British, and especially an English, ex-soldier
in such a capacity. They are always grumblers
and usually insubordinate, and their bad moral
example much more than counterbalances such
physical instruction as they may impart. After new
soldiers truly pass out of the recruit stage this vigilance may be relaxed, and at no time should concern
degenerate into friction and worry. Perpetual nag-
ging—too curious supervision—is almost as bad as
contemptuous neglect.

Where water is scarce, a very small quantity, a
quart, with a small sponge or a damp towel is sufficient for cleanliness. Where it is abundant, plunge
bathing should be encouraged, except in the very
heat of the day or near nightfall. Soldiers should
be encouraged to carry a cake of soap, in a small
flannel bag to avoid waste. For officers, soap
"leaves" in a small water-proof box, to be carried

in the pocket, are most convenient. Every prolonged campaign where opportunities for the care of
the person are deficient is marked by the presence
of vermin. These may affect any grade. The odor
of musk is said to be deterrent, but it can only be
used exceptionally. To thoroughly boil the clothing or to soak it in sea-water or other brine is the
simplest way of destroying the infection. To soak
infected clothing in a barrel of water containing a
handful of "fish berries" (cocculus indicus) is said
on good authority to be efficacious. A careful captain has been known to carry these with his company
property for this especial purpose.

New soldiers invariably begin field service by
attempting to carry too much, and then very soon
they abandon necessary things. There should be prepared in advance two schedules, one of articles that
must and another of such as may be carried. The
limit of the first should not be lowered nor that of
the second be exceeded. But after six months the
second schedule may be abandoned, in view of the
experience acquired. On daily marches it is found
that washing the face and neck on rising is not well,
probably because the removal of the natural secre-
tion makes the skin more susceptible to the dust and
heat of the route. To wash the eyes and mouth
and use a damp towel on the face and neck is preferable. When camp is reached the entire body if possible, and invariably the head, the genitals and
adjacent folds, and the feet, should be washed.
Soldiers' hair should always be kept short.

When lying out of barracks, soil-dampness should
always be guarded against by an impermeable sheet,

as the rubber blanket, between the man and the ground, or the soldier should have a few inches of air-space under him. In a wooded country immediate steps should be taken to build platforms at least two and better four feet from the soil upon which the tents may rest. The natural sod should not be removed. To raise the tent thus is not difficult, and it has secured the immunity of an entire command owing to the air-swept space under the sleepers. If the tents cannot be elevated, bunks must be raised well above the ground. Even with shelter tents, there must be some approach to this. Under no circumstances should the men sleep directly on the ground, and whatever constitutes the floor, whether boards, boughs, or straw, must be removed and the surface swept and exposed to the air, and if possible to the sun, every dry day. Tent walls should not be raised to windward after nightfall. Vegetation liable to decay is not healthful to sleep upon.

Except under overruling military objections, which would rarely occur, tents should open to the east, and the southern wall be raised in good weather after the day is advanced, so that sunlight may search it throughout. Tents not on elevated platforms should be moved weekly to the alternate spaces that would remain in the lines.

Every tent should be ditched as soon as pitched. That is a good rule for all camps not in rainless regions, and an imperative one in damp places. In any climate dampness of a tent floor is harmful. On the second day at the latest, company and other streets should be prepared   These and a gen-

eral system of superficial drainage are everywhere
essential for comfort and in wet climates for health.
It by no means follows that because a command
is in the field it has an adequate air-supply. Canvas when wet is practically impermeable to the air,
and in a wooded or chapparal country there may be
little movement of the atmosphere. Camps may
readily be too compact, and troops marching in
close order are liable to modified crowd-poisoning.
The utmost extension of a camp that military considerations will permit, within the limits of reasonable
police supervision, is always necessary, and especially so in a hot country. In hot weather all tents,
shelter or other, standing more than one night should
be protected overhead by a brush canopy, and brush
arbors in front of tents should be built by the second
day. These should be arranged to protect from the
sun with the least interference with the wind. In
camps of any duration vegetable decay from these
shades must be guarded against. For camps of position portable huts or sheds may be furnished. These,
whose frames may be of wood or iron, should have
ridge ventilation from rafters crossing beyond the
true peak, louvered lateral openings in the wall, and
a steep roof to throw off the rain. Temporary huts
of the same general character with fairly open walls
can speedily be built where there is light timber.
They need not be more than 16 feet wide nor 10 feet
to the eaves. Every structure for habitation should
be ditched as carefully as the tents, and by preference be raised on posts well clear of the ground. In
cold weather it should be well banked. If the floor
is not raised, the boards should be fastened with

screws and be frequently removed. As with tents,
the principles of dry soil, a free air-space under the
floor, and abundant ventilation and sunlight should
be maintained.

Notwithstanding air may have free access, neither
barracks nor tents should be overcrowded. Consumption spreads readily under such circumstances
the world over. In all stationary camps the men
develop a tendency to accumulate useless articles.
These are hurtful by interfering with the living space,

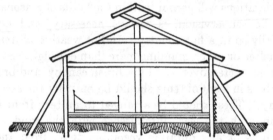

From Notter and Firth's Hygiene. (By the courtesy of Messrs. P
Blakiston & Co)

harboring dust, and sometimes promoting decay, and
should relentlessly be condemned. At every daily
inspection in dry weather the floor should be absolutely bare, and the ground beneath it be observed.

The proper police of all military camps is important, particularly in southern climates where
the combination of heat and moisture leads to the
rapid decomposition of waste and encourages the
plague of flies. Hence all refuse should be promptly
removed without the lines and everything that is
combustible be burned. Incombustible material
should be buried in trenches, partly for the sake of

order and partly that no débris in sight may serve
as an excuse for other such neglect. Kitchen waste
should be disposed of twice daily.

The sinks, miscalled latrines except when there is
water carriage, on every account require the greatest
care. They should be placed to leeward if possible,
and always no farther away than absolutely necessary, for when properly cared for they need not offend
the sense of smell or of sight. The company kitchens
and the general sinks should be on opposite sides of
the camp; for it is well estabilshed that some diseases may be communicated by flies that have alighted
in sinks transferring with their feet infected particles
of filth to prepared food in the hands of the cooks or
of the men. It is imperative that sinks should not
drain toward the water-supply. Each sink should
be from 12 to 20 ft. long by 6 to 8 or more ft. deep,
if intended for use more than twenty-four hours. It
is better to multiply the sinks than to make them
too long. In each case all the earth should be
thrown to the rear. For a single day's use 3 ft. is
deep enough. But they should be dug immediately
for every part of a command of any size. It is only
a small body of actively moving troops, that will not
be followed by others, that can afford to dispense
with them for a single night. In that case, as well
as before sinks are dug if there is even trifling delay,
a small area must be set apart to leeward where men
may relieve themselves. When this is done and the
men are equipped with an intrenching tool, each
man should be required to cover his evacuations
with fresh earth immediately. The use of sinks or of
a limited locality should be strictly enforced. There

is no more distinct sign of ill-disciplined troops than
the soil pollution that follows such neglect. Sinks
should be screened by bushes and be covered from
the sun when possible. In very wet seasons old
canvas may be reserved to protect in part from
the rain. Under the same conditions the excavated
earth should be kept dry as far as may be. Enough
dry earth to completely cover the deposits should
be thrown in evenly at least thrice daily—at retreat,
after breakfast, and at noon. If lime can be pro-
cured it should be added if there is the least evidence
of dysentery in the command, for dysentery may be
contracted by the well who frequent foul latrines
used by such sick. To burn a little mineral oil on
paper or straw thrown into the sink helps to keep
down the flies. When within two feet of the surface
the sink should be filled in, rounded over, distinctly
marked, and a new one prepared in the same general neighborhood. All sinks should be filled in on
breaking camp and all débris burned, if there is no
military objection to the smoke from the fires. Officers' sinks should have box seats open to the rear,
and be well protected in front, rear, and overhead.
Urinals should be arranged in convenient places in a
camp of permanence, and their use compelled; for it is
perfectly possible to communicate such a disease as
typhoid fever by urine indiscriminately voided. The
sinks used by the sick are to be disinfected as the
medical officer may direct, and all sinks are to be
inspected daily by the officer of the day in addition
to the medical officer's inspection.

Cheerfulness is absolutely necessary for a healthy
camp. The two elements that insure this are occu-

pation and amusement. *Ennui* is the parent of discontent and homesickness. Discontent spoils the best soldier, and homesickness is a most depressing disease. Regular occupation besides drills is necessary. After a camp is well established work, preferably of a military character should be found, as for instance the making of field defences, or of gabions and fascines. This should not be carried to exhaustion, nor occupy all the spare time. At the same time athletic games should be encouraged and if necessary be organized and contests arranged. One of the tests of an officer's fitness for his commission is his ability to interest his men in such matters. Music is always stimulating, and martial music is a great solace in the discomfort of the field. Gambling, to which many men will resort in the absence of rational amusement, is hurtful physically and morally. It tends to keep men out of the fresh air in crowded groups and constrained positions, it encourages nearly all of the baser emotions, and is a great obstacle to discipline in peace or war. When circumstances permit, short marches, especially with all the forms of war, are exciting and instructive. Commendatory orders by the brigade and regimental commanders for the neatest regimental camps and company streets, and for the regiment and company freest from preventable disease, encourage the better men. This principle of commendation is applicable to divisions and corps.

There are two great classes of diseases, the intestinal and the malarial, that threaten and generally afflict an army in the field in the warmer climates, and in the American tropics a third, yellow fever,

that is greatly to be dreaded. All of these are preventable in the sense of. being avoidable. The
exposures of field life are often followed by their
attacks, but they frequently occur because perfectly
practicable precautions have been neglected. These
will first be considered, and then general rules for
preserving health, in addition to those already laid
down for the care of camps, will be added.

The intestinal diseases proper that befall an army,
especially in the South, are temporary looseness of
the bowels, a debilitating and persistent diarrhœa,
and dysentery, acute and chronic, always serious
and often dangerous. These all may occur in succession in the same person. Typhoid fever, which is
apt to invade and to spread in ill-kept camps, has its
main seat in the bowels and is propagated by their
discharges. All these are avoidable by mature and
healthy men; or, more strictly, they only occur after
violation of personal or general hygiene. The cau-
tions to be observed by line officers in these respects
in the care of those under them are as follows:

Malarial infection weakens the natural powers of
resistance and may complicate any of the diseases
mentioned. There is therefore a particular reason
for guarding against it, as will presently be
described.

As popularly recognized, errors of diet are a common cause of diarrhœa. Recruits often suffer from
diarrhœa even in garrison, simply because of unaccustomed food; and all but seasoned men are liable
to it when the conditions of camp cooking are first
encountered. If the food itself is sound and is properly prepared, this will soon pass away. But careful

and intelligent supervision of the kitchens and the mess is necessary.

Water quite free from specific disease-causes may induce diarrhœa, that may become very serious in susceptible persons. Hard water, chiefly from lime and magnesium salts, may be modified by boiling. But generally speaking, the system becomes habituated to it, especially if it is drank sparingly at first. To drink from alluvial rivers filled with suspended clay will induce diarrhœa in unaccustomed persons, and sometimes in all. Such water will frequently become clear by merely standing for twenty-four hours (sedimentation). Filtering slowly through flannel detains much of the mud, but the flannel must frequently be changed or washed. Chopped cactus-leaves have a clarifying effect, and an excellent agent is alum, in the proportion of six grains to the gallon, stirred in the water to carry the clay down as a precipitate. Some such precaution is necessary with the water of muddy rivers. Occasionally it is found that water charged with vegetable débris causes diarrhœa, but is harmless when filtered. Brackish water from near the sea may cause diarrhœa, when the only preventive would be distillation. The same is true of alkaline water. An effective distilling apparatus can be constructed by the aid of a kerosene lamp, a small metal tank, a few feet of pipe, and a receiving vessel. (*See figure.*) This is not nearly as complicated as it appears, and is very portable and inexpensive. *P* and *S*, stands, can be extemporized in any camp.

For permanent posts, when required, the Quartermaster's Department will supply distilling apparatus on a large scale, and for camps where the water is doubtful porcelain filters are furnished. The latter are fragile and need great care in their management and transportation. Practicable filters of sand and gravel in casks can be extemporized in the field.

One but not the sole cause of dysentery, very serious and very common in the tropics, is water polluted with excremental matter, and particularly

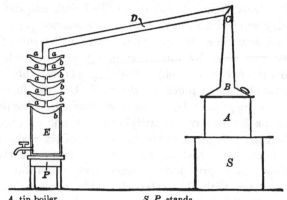

A, tin boiler.
B, tin funnel-top.
C, sleeve of 2-in. pipe *D*.
E, jar, preferably earthen.

S, P, stands.
ab, condensing plates, pressed tin.
a, one inch deep; *b*, three inches deep.

A 1-inch tube 3 inches long is soldered to the top of *a*, and a tube 2 inches long, to slide into the other, is soldered to the bottom of *b*.
If *A* is 17 inches square each perpendicular inch will contain one gallon.
From the design of Major Alfred E. Sears, by the courtesy of The Medical Record.

with the discharges from a previous case. Once introduced it is liable to become epidemic; hence special pains should be taken to guard the water from the very beginning, to avoid old camp-grounds, and occasionally to occupy a new site. Where the purity of the water is maintained, much freedom from this disease is assured. Where the water is impure or even doubtful, every drop drank or used with food should be boiled, whether in camp or while marching. With fairly disciplined troops this is perfectly feasible.

Both typhoid fever and dysentery may, however, be propagated by minute particles of excreta, or the bacteria from them, attached to food or driven as dust into the mouth. Hence scrupulous police care should be enforced within the habitable limits of the camp and upon its confines. It is certain that the painless diarrhœa of the unrecognized first stage of true typhoid fever is infective. Therefore these are reasons additional to those of abstract cleanliness for the careful control of all evacuations.

Tropical dysentery is very persistent and readily reasserts itself. A convalescent therefrom is not fit for the field until long after he seems to be well. Typhoid fever disqualifies a soldier for at least three months, on account of changes in some of the inner organs. Company officers should always be prepared to lose the services of such men for prolonged periods.

The malarial diseases are represented by the intermittent fevers, from the common ague to the crushing pernicious or congestive chill that destroys life at a single blow; by the remittent or bilious fevers, from those familiar to most residents of the central states to the Chagres and jungle fevers of the tropics; and by complications of various other well-known diseases. In the tropics these are most prevalent in the spring and autumn, the maximum coinciding with the close of the rainy season.

The efficient cause of malarial disease is a plasmodium which, in various forms, infects the blood.

This has not yet been isolated outside of the human body, except in a genus of the mosquito (*anopheles*) which acts as an intermediate host and transfers it from man to man. This is a demonstrated fact, and completely accounts for all the presumed methods of its spread formerly accepted, except possibly its absorption in drinking water. Those most susceptible to its action are the weary, hungry, and ill-conditioned, and those weakened by excesses. If the possibility of drinking infected water be rejected, and there is no positive evidence that the disease may be communicated in that way, the prevention of malaria in the field is summed up in the exclusion of the mosquito. In its final expression this is by the use of nets or of some deterrent application. Contributing measures are such as these: In selecting a dry site for a camp; in encamping to the windward of marshes; in avoiding unnecessary exposure after the sun sets and until it has well risen; in being reasonably clothed, especially during sleep, with light woollen or merino, or at least loosely-woven cotton; in having the floor of the tent or sleeping-place raised several feet from the ground, which is practicable in permanent camps, and is important, but is rarely done; in drinking only water that has been boiled, which is particularly important and easily arranged; in supplying the men on night duty with hot food, such as oatmeal gruel, early in the evening, and with hot coffee and hard bread near midnight and again near dawn; and in the systematic preventive use of quinine for those particularly exposed, and c curative doses on the slightest suspicion of a malarial invasion. All of these precau-

tions cannot be taken in the immediate presence of
the enemy, against whom military operations of
attack or defence may be of primary importance;
but it is astonishing how much that is preventive
may be done ordinarily by systematic and intelligent
forethought. The delay of a few nights in a highly
malarious region may weaken an army more than
a sharp engagement. Even where the locality is
not "pernicious" in the technical sense, prolonged
residence in an unhealthy situation depresses the
men physically and morally by the resulting sickness.
and death. For instance, it is probable that the
Army of the Potomac, notwithstanding it compelled
a bloodless evacuation, lost more men during the
month it lay in front of Yorktown in the spring of
1862, and subsequently as a consequence of that
camp, than would have fallen under an immediate
assault.

Other precautions that always may be taken are:
Every soldier may wear a light woollen suit next
to the skin. That is a matter of equipment first and
of discipline afterward. It is useless to supply men
with heavy woollen underwear in a hot climate and
to expect it to be worn. It becomes insufferable,
and will be abandoned or destroyed. The temptation with ill-disciplined troops is to do the same even
with very light flannel; but, partly by explanation
and partly by rigid discipline, they may be held to it
until it is worn willingly. Its habitual use, especially at night, relieves the body from the risk of
debilitating chill.

To drink only water that has been well and comparatively recently boiled. Water for a company

may be boiled wherever a camp-kettle can be carried; and every man can boil his own allowance whenever he can make an individual fire for his own cup. A zealous captain will see that his men actually fill their canteens with boiled water before they fall in for the march, and that while in camp or bivouac they drink none that is raw. Well-made tea (where water that has boiled must be used) or boiled coffee is still more acceptable, and men should be encouraged to carry tea or coffee (in a vial for economy) and to boil the water in their own cups on making camp. A canteen of tea is more desirable than one of plain water. The object in drinking only boiled water is the exclusion of any other depressing pollution, quite regardless of the possible presence of the malarial plasmodium or its antecedent. But "it is regarded as not impossible that the drinking of water contaminated by these insects [mosquitoes] . . . may have a part in the dissemination" [of malarial fever]. (Harrington.) To boil the water devitalizes the plasmodium.

When deprived of the conveniences of camp, as here supposed, preventive doses of quinine should not only be dispensed but administered, and that *without* whiskey. It is as absurd to campaign within range of malaria without using quinine as it would be to go into battle without ammunition. But the use of alcohol before or during such exposure opens the system to its attack. Hot and tolerably strong coffee is an excellent tonic under such conditions.

The foregoing represents nearly everything that can be done under those emergencies which compel active movements in malarial tracts.

Yellow fever is now believed to be transmitted
from man to man by the agency of the mosquito
(*Stegomyia fasciata*), precisely as the malarial disease is spread by the *anopheles*. It is not known to
be propagated in any other way, and the disease-cause
has not yet been discovered outside of man and this
insect. Hence protection from it consists in avoiding the infected mosquito, and its prevention is concerned with destroying, primarily, all the insects
thus contaminated and, secondarily, those capable
of becoming an intermediate host. The Army Commission under Major Reed appears to have determined definitely that everything outside of these living bodies may be disregarded. The incubation in
man does not exceed five days. Therefore any well
man may be admitted from an infected district without fear after that period of isolation has elapsed. The
infected mosquito requires twelve days for the infection to develop. It follows that all mosquitoes that
have not been in contact with a yellow-fever case for
a little more than twelve days are harmless. But
once infected, it is believed that the insect may cause
the disease for an almost indefinite time, certainly
after a period of prolonged hibernation. In the field
yellow fever, having occurred, will ravage a non-
immune command while it remains where the disease appeared. Ultimate military success will therefore best be attained by effectually avoiding places
known to be infected. Even in the tropics the
removal of an infected command from bodies of
water and to a height of 1000 feet will often check
the epidemic. In more temperate climates to trans-
fer the troops, frequently only twenty or thirty

miles, into a drier and somewhat higher atmosphere
will generally cause the disease to cease. In both
cases presumably this is because the *Stegomyia* does
not breed there, although such local exemption has
not yet been demonstrated. Should the command
remain stationary after the disease appears, every
man who has not previously had it will certainly be
attacked as long as infecting mosquitoes can reach
him. The accession of frost sets the only natural
limitation to their ravages. The mortality from
yellow fever is always high, and men broken by
excess, especially alcoholics, almost certainly succumb when attacked. It is the true policy, whenever practicable, to manœuvre oneself out of and the
enemy into the yellow-fever region. Both malarial-
and yellow-fever cases are always to be regarded as
infecting centres, not to be avoided by the well for
fear of direct infection, but to be protected by netting
and otherwise from those insects that imbibe, develop, and transmit such infection.

Independently of specific causes of diseases as
noted above, there are other avoidable conditions
which frequently lead to illness in warm climates.
One of the most important is the effect of heat and
cold, and particularly changes from one to the other,
in causing diarrhœa and dysentery. Men become
chilled at night, or by the evaporation of perspiration after exertion, when the bowels soon suffer.
Systematic attention to so simple a matter as insuring
that men are properly covered at night is important.
Young soldiers, and particularly those unaccustomed to camp, cannot be depended upon to care
for themselves, but the captain who makes sure that

his men *are* thus protected will be certain of a stronger and more willing command. The bowels lie so near the wall of the abdomen that the circulation there, on whose disturbance this form of diarrhœa primarily depends, is easily deranged by changes of temperature.

The cummerbund of the Asiatics and the cholera belt of Eastern travellers, evolved by experience, are intended to equalize the abdominal circulation. More convenient than these and more efficient is a flannel apron, of one or two thicknesses, from 14 to 18 inches in width and from 6 to 8 in depth, tied by a tape around the waist and worn directly next the skin. This apron is quite different from the official belt that has been issued, which is apt, when it is unwillingly worn, to become an ineffectual and annoying roll about the waist. It lies in place, is easily tolerated, and generally prevents or controls the simple diarrhœa or light dysentery of either hot or cold climates that depends upon disturbances of the local circulation. The apron is not issued by the government, but it is procurable, and every commanding officer in hot climates should insist that his men are provided with two apiece, and should verify by irregular inspections that one of them is constantly worn. To some officers such attention to the individual men as is implied in these paragraphs does not appeal. But to those who remember how frequently soldiers are exposed to illness, partly from ignorance and partly from helplessness, this form of duty becomes a pleasure that meets a most effectual reward.

One of the direct effects of extreme heat is sunstroke, or heat-exhaustion, and when high temperature is long continued there is a general depression quite independent of such direct causes as the malarial or other poisons. The head covering should be light in weight and in color, be permeable to the air, and have an air-space all around as well as above the head. When directly exposed to the sun, a wet sponge or wet muslin worn in the crown lessens the risk. Experience shows that the second great nervous centre, the spinal cord, should not be exposed directly to the sun for a length of time. All the clothing should be loose, especially about the neck and chest, and the pack that may require to be borne should stand away from the body. The general depression from long-continued heat is intensified in a moist climate by imperfect ventilation.

As the companies fall in for a march or similar duty, inspection of canteens should show them filled with pure water, preferably boiled, or weak tea. In temperate climates men should be discouraged from drinking en route. Once begun, the almost irresistible temptation is to drink frequently and then to replenish the canteen from the nearest water regardless of quality. The sensation of ordinary thirst arises from dryness of the fauces, and if these are moistened by the saliva excited by chewing there is great relief. To that end it is better to supply the system by a reasonable draught of water before starting, and to keep a pebble or a bit f wood in the mouth to excite moisture, but not to drink a drop, except there may be a halt for luncheon, until the camp for the day is in sight. In the tropics this rule must be somewhat modified, for too great loss of fluid by perspiration predisposes to heat prostration, and a part of the liquid must be replaced. But whatever is drank while marching should be limited in amount and be taken at considerable intervals, and the men should be particularly cautioned against drinking much early on the way. Exact and arbitrary control over the use of the canteen is impracticable and would be unwise, but through their noncommissioned officers the privates must constantly be instructed, until from reason and experience the habit of abstinence is acquired and they learn that tropical water must be boiled.

But, as Smart points out, under a blazing tropical sun a fulminant heat-stroke is better avoided by using a stinted but steady supply than by drinking copiously with a period of enforced abstinence following.

The question of diet in an unaccustomed climate is a vexed one. It is a good general rule to follow the habits of intelligent natives without changing too suddenly from the usual food. All food in hot climates is prone to decay, but nothing should be eaten that is open to suspicion. Natives frequently consume decomposing food with impunity, and in that respect their example is not to be followed. When ripe and perfectly sound, fruit is generally unobjectionable; but within the tropics the least spot upon it indicating decay should condemn the whole. The difficulty of enforcing this rule with soldiers leads to the more general one of forbidding all fruit. This is not a necessity, but is an effort to avoid a frequent evil.

Alcohol in any form and to any degree as a beverage is harmful, and when taken beyond moderation is dangerous. It is true the world over that a drunken camp is a sickly camp, and in hot climates drinking, even short of excess, tends directly to disease.

Properly to conduct a march requires experience, or a greater attention to theory than frequently is given. Except the necessity be very pressing, the first march with troops unseasoned in marching, however well they may be drilled otherwise, should be but a very few miles, barely enough to clear the old camps, for at the outset there is friction everywhere. Each day's march may be gradually increased until in about a fortnight the maximum will be reached. By this gradual development much better results can be secured in a given time than would be were a specified distance equally divided through a given number of days. Every eight or ten days besides Sundays there should be a halt for rest and repairs. Under pressure seasoned infantry will make almost incredible distances and great speed, as witness Crawfurd's Light Division in the Peninsular War and "Stonewall" Jackson's command in our Civil War. Enthusiastic cavalrymen are unwilling to admit it, but it appears true that seasoned infantry will outmarch mounted troops in a long compaign. Good marching is the complement of good fighting, and the most famous and effective troops are those that reach the objective the soonest; but no troops can march their best until they are taught. The ease with which troops march is inversely to the size of the command; thus a regiment moves more easily than a division, a division better than a corps. Over good roads fourteen miles in ten hours is good marching for a large army, but a regiment will easily make that distance in four hours including halts. Infantry and mounted troops should not march together if it can be avoided, and infantry should march with as wide a front and in as open order as possible, for crowd-poisoning follows the collection of dirty, heated men out of doors as well as within houses. After the first few regiments, troops almost invariably march in dust or mud, and close order is very distressing. With a large command, if it is possible to move troops in columns parallel to the roads so as to leave these free for the trains, it should always be done, for it is a great comfort to have the wagons at hand when camp is made. Unless the command is very small, the men should be required to pay no attention to the minor obstacles of mud, water, and the like; for hesitation in the leading files is magnified into serious halts at the rear, and a jerky progress is very trying. But it is an economy of time to have fallen trees that partly obstruct the way entirely removed. Under the best circumstances even good troops will lose distance, and frequent halts are necessary or the rear will be in a state of perpetual worry in the effort to close up. No particular command should be moved on until it is well closed up in the rear and the rear ranks have rested. The first halt would better be at the end of half an hour, and be used by the men in relieving themselves and adjusting their clothes and their burdens. There should be a halt for five or ten minutes (as prescribed) at the end of every subsequent hour, when the men should be encouraged to spread out and rest, but never be allowed to straggle from the column for any purpose. The length of all occasional halts when foreseen should be announced at the beginning and passed down the column, for uncertainty destroys much of the benefit of the rest. Even in those accidental stops that occur in every column, should the regimental or other commanders take pains to discover the probable delay and communicate it by special signal in order that the men might rest, their strength and temper would be much conserved. Few conditions are more trying to men under arms than to await on their feet an uncertain advance. The French use a device to save time in resuming the march and to keep the men out of the mud, where squads of twenty or thirty form a circle and each man sits on the knees of the man in rear. At formal halts to get the full advantage of rest the men should lie flat on their backs with their belts loosened, but with a poncho or some other protection between their bodies and damp ground.

Straggling, the loitering behind of the sick, the tired, the lazy, the ill-disciplined, is an evil indirectly affecting the health and the *morale*, and directly concerning the military vigor of the column. Its prevention, so far as those out of health are concerned, depends upon the prompt and rigid scrutiny by the medical officers of all who fall out claiming to be sick and their immediate disposition. All not adjudged sick should be promptly returned to the ranks or, in common with the other stragglers, be taken in charge by the provost guard. It is better that those really unfit should be provided with a formal ticket describing them, naming their presumed disability and distinctly defining from what they are excused. Such details, however, may safely be left to the administration of the medical department. But any man out of ranks without the written permission of his company commander on a prearranged card should be assumed a straggler, unless showing *prima facie* evidence of illness. Men fairly tired out will often be brought up fresh at the end of a few hours' transportation, but this privilege is so liable to abuse that it should rarely be given. But the really ill are to be carefully carried, for with good troops one should take the most thoughtful care of them, because then they will put forth their best efforts in the belief that they will be protected and restored when disabled. For this reason, among others, it is important that its ambulance-train should immediately follow each division. Under exceptional circumstances one or more ambulances should accompany each brigade.

The music of the fife and drum is of material assistance to a tired column, and even the steady drum tap alone helps the pace of the weary. The men should always be encouraged to sing on the march, for the more cheerful a command the more easily it moves.

It is usually an error to break camp before day, as is sometimes done, and night marches are to be avoided if possible. In non-malarious regions in hot weather an occasional night march under a light moon is a relief, but as a rule the loss of sleep and the general discomfort thus caused outbalance any ordinary advantage. Should a military necessity compel a night march in a malarious region, a preventive dose of quinine ought to be administered to every one involved, as would be done in other night duty.

In a very hot climate marches should be so regulated that the sun may not shine directly on the men's backs, because extreme heat on the spinal column is harmful. This is important and frequently has been neglected.

In conclusion, it must always be remembered that men abruptly transferred from civil life to the field have new and artificial circumstances to which to adapt themselves, and in proportion as their own freedom of action is restrained does the responsibility of the officers in direct command increase. That responsibility is not limited to instruction in drill, but runs, coequal with their authority, over every condition and detail of military life. The care of troops is a serious and constant matter of daily duty, which may be neglected but cannot be evaded; and as a rule the proportion of men presenting themselves as sick is an index of the intelligence and fidelity with which that duty is discharged. For, reduced to its final expression, the efficiency of a command is measured by the intelligent care that has been bestowed upon it.

X.

ADDENDA.

Asepsis as Applied to Wounds.

In addition to the mechanical injury inflicted by a bullet, the wound is liable to inflammation and discharge. That was formerly regarded as necessary after gunshot. It is now known that the inflammation is incited by the presence of infinitesimal forms of life called bacteria. These prevail on the surface of all substances, animate and inanimate, not made aseptic by special treatment, and invariably are introduced in wounds when probed or handled on the field. If they are excluded, most wounds not fatal in themselves can be treated successfully. But usually wounds become infected before a medical officer sees them. It is of the utmost importance for the men to understand that there should be no interference even with the surface of any wound, but that it should be immediately covered with the preventive dressing that every soldier carries. If that is done at once, and the hand, the clothing, and other foreign matters are kept away, there is a fair prospect of recovery in those cases that are not by their very nature and degree immediately fatal. This doctrine of non-interference and of aseptic dressing should be taught at every opportunity.

The first-aid packet, which is part of the equip-

ment of every soldier, contains all that is necessary
for the immediate care of any wound that is not complicated with severe hæmorrhage or with the fracture
of a large bone. The experience of late wars shows
that not only much surgical illness and suffering
have been avoided, but many lives have been saved,
by the immediate application of those dressings as
directed, and by abstention from interference before
or afterward. Foreign bodies are kept out, so that
the natural processes of healing begin and go on
without interruption. The results expected to follow that simple procedure are so remarkable that
the average soldier is incredulous that they will
occur. He thinks that something more should be
done at the time, and he fails to recognize the importance of the plain instruction to apply these
sterilized dressings and to abstain from meddling.
On this account the primary treatment and the
consecutive non-interference should be a matter of
formal and peremptory military precept from the
company officers, as well as of general explanation
from the medical officers.

The natural ignorance on the soldier's part of the
real value of the first-aid packets, and his scep-
ticism as to their importance even when that is explained, as well perhaps as the readiness with which
they are replaced gratuitously when lost or destroyed,
lead him to think lightly of keeping them intact, or
indeed of keeping them at all. They are acceptable
as wash-cloths and convenient for gun-rags, and
where there is not reasonable discipline very many
of them are wasted in that way. Besides, enormous
numbers have been spoiled in tropical field service

through humidity and by friction against other objects. When the moderately water-proof covering is damaged, the usefulness of the packet is diminished if not estroyed. The remedy is not merely to assign the packet to a defined position in a proper receptacle, so that it will always be carried by the man in the same place and may be found readily, but also to hold the soldier to the same responsibility for it that he has for other public property, and to verify its presence and its good condition by frequent formal inspections. When the soldier habitually regards it as public property for which there is accountability, and not as a personal perquisite, he will pay it more respect.

SCHEME FOR A SANITARY INSPECTION BY COMPANY OFFICERS.

In Garrison.

Squad-room: Capacity and permissible number of occupants according to the sanitary standard. Number who slept in the squad-room last night. Maximum number present at any time since last inspection, with date.

Floor-space per bunk.

Air-space per occupant, disregarding height above 14 feet and taking account of objects in the apartment.

Illumination, natural: Arrangement and sufficiency.

Illumination, artificial: Method; number of lights; sufficiency for comfort; influence upon the air.

Sunlight: Does direct sunlight reach all parts of the room at some time of the day? If not, explain.

Heating: Method; relation to comfort of inmates; to air, by escape of CO or otherwise.

Ventilation: Style and sufficiency. Observe carefully at irregular intervals, and especially at night, whether the openings remain unobstructed. Is the whole room air-swept daily?

Odor: Note the degree of odor, if any, soon after midnight and again before dawn, and the state of the ventilating apparatus then.

Bunks and bedding: Inspect minutely some particular bunk for general cleanliness, and especially for freedom from vermin; inspect several for objects under the pillow or mattress, as soiled clothes, food, tobacco. Examine the under side of an occasional mattress for dust. How frequently and completely is the bedding exposed out of doors?

Cuspidors: Kind, number, and condition.

Floors: Are they clean and dry? How are they habitually cleansed? Are they ever damp?

Walls and ceilings: Are they clean and unstained by smoke or otherwise? When were they lime-washed, or they and the woodwork painted? Examine corners, the tops of the lower sashes, and behind boxes.

Lockers: Examine, not merely for order, but for dust or dirt and odor.

Clothing not on the person: Is the uniform clean? Is the underclothing clean, or properly set apart for the wash? Examine carefully the soles of spare shoes. No shoe should bring in dirt from out of doors.

Clothing on the person: Open the coats, examine the shirt, undershirt, and the surface of the chest; examine one foot bare and the stocking on the other foot; expose and inspect the lower part of the drawers; are the head and neck and the inside of the cap clean? are the hair and beard closely trimmed? (Excuse non-commissioned officers from this personal inspection.)

Flies: If there are many flies, determine the reason. (Flies imply the presence of organic débris.)

Mosquitoes: Are there adequate nets? Are they used?

At a formal inspection insist that everything commonly in the squad-room is in place. Allow neither necessary nor extra articles to be hidden— "put away on account of inspection."

Examine every occupied room, especially those of the cooks if they sleep out of the squad-room, in the same manner.

Examine attic and general store-rooms cursorily, to see that no improper articles, as food or soiled clothes, are concealed there.

Mess-room: Examine it and the table furniture,

including the under side of the table if it is reversible, for cleanliness. Inspect carefully the insides of the bowls and the tines of the forks. Examine also table furniture not actually upon the table, and the floors and windows, all for cleanliness.

Water-coolers and pitchers: Examine the interiors carefully, wherever found.

Kitchen: The interior of all cooking utensils should be scrupulously clean. Examine floors, walls, tables, and plumbing, including grease trap, if any. Knives, cleavers, strainers, should be free from débris. Examine the interior of refrigerator daily. Inspect for roaches about range and slop-sink. Examine all food, whether cooking or in store. Especially in hot climates, see that no food is decomposing. Observe carefully the presence of flies.

Cellar: Inspect for dryness, ventilation, freedom from odor, and for condition of contents.

Grounds: Inspect those immediately around the barracks and under the verandas, as for general police and for dryness. Where there is no cellar, determine the condition under the building.

Garbage barrels or boxes: How frequently, how completely, and in what manner is the garbage disposed of? Is the neighboring ground polluted? Follow up in detail the disposal of waste.

Sinks and urinals: What disposition is made of body waste? Inspect carefully and frequently for interior and exterior cleanliness. If the sinks or urinals give out odor, ascertain the cause and present a remedy. If urine is voided in unauthorized places, determine the fact and stop it.

Wash-room: Number and condition of basins, overflow, and floors.

Bathing facilities: Examine for sufficiency, for cleanliness, and for frequency of use. Be satisfied that every soldier not sick bathes completely at stated intervals, and that the tubs are clean.

Waste water: Where there is no sewerage, what is its disposition?

Guard-house: Capacity, cleanliness, ventilation, heating, and number of occupants of cells and of prison room separately. Prisoners may properly be uncomfortable, but their health should not be allowed to suffer in the least.

Guard-room: The guard should not be unnecessarily uncomfortable and their apartment should be well ventilated, not unduly warm, and entirely free from gross dirt. There should be facilities for preparing a hot luncheon for the reliefs going on post at and after midnight. All these points should be observed. Clothing and blankets, whether of the guard or of prisoners, should be inspected or treated for vermin before being re-introduced into the barracks.

Stables: Ventilation, light, and relation of windows to horses. Is the floor dry? If sickness among horses, examine for soil-moisture and, if necessary, recommend deep drainage. If flies are numerous, determine the cause. Note the disposition of liquid waste within and of the general manure without the stables. (Peat moss for bedding prevents ammoniacal odor in the stalls.)

Married men's quarters: Inspect every room for air-space, ventilation, light, and general cleanliness. Inspect the cellar, if any, for dampness and odor. Observe carefully the disposition of kitchen waste and of laundry slops.

Privies: In those posts or parts of posts where there is no sewage, the privies must be carefully supervised by the companies responsible, and every one should be inspected once a week. Where they are pits they should be filled with fresh earth when within two feet of the surface, marked, and reported to the quartermaster to be noted on the post map. No pit for this purpose should be dug without authority from the commanding officer. The vicinity of stables, corrals, wood-piles, haystacks, should be carefully inspected for superficial pollution. Each company must carefully guard against contaminating a local water-supply.

In the Field.

Follow as far as applicable the form for garrison inspection. Also:

Tents: Character; number of inmates; ditched? Whether floored or not floored, is the ground dry and clean? How much above the floor is the bunk? Is the canvas sound? How ventilated, heated? How frequently removed to new site? If not regularly moved, how frequently struck? Are the walls raised daily in fair weather? In the warm season, to leeward at night? Is unauthorized material, particularly food, present? In a malarious region do the men have nets, and use them?

Huts: Material; size; shape; cubic capacity; mode of heating; ventilation; lighting; condition of floor; style of bunks; unauthorized material, especially food, present; water-tight or not; dry or damp; ditched and banked; sickness since last inspection; lateral distance between huts; distance to next in rear?

Company street: Is it of proper width; well tamped; ditched; dusty; muddy; well policed?

Kitchen: Cleanliness of ground, tables, utensils. How is food protected before cooking; after? Distance from kitchen sink; distance from nearest part of company street; direction and distance from company sinks; prevailing wind; do flies appear to reach the kitchen from company sink, directly or otherwise? Direct disposition of waste from kitchen.

Mess table: If such a table, condition of it and the adjacent ground; are flies there, excepting when meals are served; how are individual utensils cleansed? If no mess table, is food eaten at the tents or at the kitchen? If at the tents, are remains of food found there?

Kitchen sink: Character; ultimate disposition of waste; condition of surrounding ground; is it flooded by rain or from ground-water; is it treated with lime or any other disinfectant?

Company sink: Situation as to distance and direction from the nearest company street and company kitchen, with prevailing wind. Character; length; depth; protection from sun, rain, observation? How frequently and how effectively is earth thrown in? What other disinfectants, if any, introduced? What action is taken against flies, and how frequently? Recommendation. (Such sinks should be covered in and marked before breaking camp, and when their contents approach the level of the surface.)

Camp urinals: How placed in relation to company streets; how arranged; how cared for; are there signs of urination elsewhere?

Food: Variety; amount; regularity of supply; condition when issued; how cooked; waste before or after serving; sufficiency or insufficiency of any particular part of the ration?

Water-supply: How obtained by the men; how is the company supply preserved; if it appears to affect the health of the men, how; if boiling has been ordered, is any drank raw; is there deficiency; is there waste; if filtered by or for the company, how and how effectively?

The soldier: Are his uniform and equipment sufficient in amount and character; is there spare underclothing; an extra pair of stockings; do the shoes really fit (the officer should satisfy himself); are the feet in good condition (inspect); if feet not in good condition, fix responsibility and report it; is the person clean; the underclothing clean; hair and beard cropped close; is the canteen occasionally boiled and the inside always kept clean?

For the march: Again inspect the feet; inspect the kit and reject everything not authorized; inspect canteen and allow nothing but pure water (boiled in the tropics) or weak tea, and explain its proper use; inspect for abdominal apron in hot or

cold weather; in the tropics require a wet cloth or
sponge in the hat; in hot weather authorize outer
garments to be well opened when marching in route
step or at ease, to facilitate evaporation from the
body and to diminish risk of heat exhaustion. At
halts, men when fatigued should be cautioned to lie
at full length if the ground permits, or, sitting, to
lean entirely relaxed against a tree or similar support.

USEFUL BOOKS OF REFERENCE.

(In each case the latest edition.)

Growth of the Recruit and Young Soldier.   Sir Wm. Aitken.
Epitome of Tripler's Manual.   Col. C. R. Greenleaf.
Anatomy, Physiology, and Hygiene.   Dr. Jerome Walker.
The Human Body (School edition), Dr. H. N. Martin.
Soldier's Pocket-book.   Lord Wolseley.
Theory and Practice of Hygiene.   Notter and Firth.
Handbook of Hygiene.   Major A. M. Davies, R.A.M.C.
Practical Hygiene.   Dr. Charles Harrington.
Military Hygiene.   Capt. E. L. Munson.
Chemistry of Cookery.   M. Williams.
Healthy Foundations for Houses.   Glenn Brown.
How to Drain a House.   G. E. Waring, Jr.
House Drainage and Sanitary Plumbing.   W. P. Gerhard.
Rural Hygiene.   Dr. G. V. Poore.
Sanitary Engineering; Sewerage.   Baldwin Latham.
Principles of Ventilation and Heating.   Dr. J. S. Billings.
Water-supply.   W. Ripley Nichols.
Water-supply.   W. P. Mason.

INDEX.

238   INDEX.

Printed in the United States
By Bookmasters